W9-BKM-321

PREPARING
FOR
PARENTHOOD

Also by Dr. Lee Salk

The Psychology of Adjustment

How to Raise a Human Being
(with Rita Kramer)

*What Every Child Would Like
His Parents to Know*

PREPARING FOR PARENTHOOD

Understanding Your Feelings About Pregnancy, Childbirth, and Your Baby

DR. LEE SALK

Director, Division of Pediatric Psychology
The New York Hospital – Cornell Medical Center

DAVID McKAY COMPANY, INC.
New York

PREPARING FOR PARENTHOOD

COPYRIGHT © 1974 by Lee Salk

All rights reserved, including the right to re-
produce this book, or parts thereof, in any form,
except for the inclusion of brief quotations in a
review.

LIBRARY OF CONGRESS CATALOG CARD NUMBER: 74–14389
ISBN 0-679-50488-5
MANUFACTURED IN THE UNITED STATES OF AMERICA
Designed by Evelyn O'Connor

I dedicate this book to all children, everywhere, first among them, my son, Eric, and my daughter, Pia.

Author's Note

An author interested in eliminating sexism from his or her work is immediately confronted with the masculine traditions of the English language. I personally reject the practice of using masculine pronouns to refer to human beings. Accordingly I have freely alternated my references, sometimes using the female gender and sometimes using the male gender.

Acknowledgments

I have particularly enjoyed working with my editor and close friend, Dan Catlin. Our friendship has grown during our work together on this book and my previous one. Dan and his wife, Dundeen, share my intense interest in the welfare of children. The dedicated father of four sons, Dan has helped guide me, not only editorially but by sharing his experience as a father and as a warm and sensitive human being. When we are together, our casual conversation generally leads to ideas for using new ways to communicate essential information to parents.

My two hardworking assistants, Nancy Raisor Schlossberg and Jenny Mlawsky, contributed most generously and selflessly helped in the metamorphosis of ideas into printed words. For this I am most grateful.

Notable among the nursing staff in the parenthood-education program who work closely with me in the new parent classes of the Lying-In Division of The New York Hospital–Cornell Medical Center are Fritzi Kallop and Dorothy Metzger. Their knowledge and their sensitivity

ACKNOWLEDGMENTS

to the problems of new parents has been effectively shared with countless people.

Finally, I would like to express my gratitude
to my friends and colleagues in the International
Childbirth Education Association and the
American National Red Cross who transmit my
ideas in their classes. They highlighted the need
for this book and encouraged me to communicate my philosophy as widely as possible in our
joint interest—preparing parents for parenthood.

Contents

PREPARING
FOR
PARENTHOOD

–I–

Your Mixed Feelings About Becoming a Parent

Taking parenthood for granted can have disastrous effects. People can and do become parents without any awareness whatsoever of the deep responsibilities, as well as the joys, the worries, and the tremendous effort that parenthood requires. Now that you are into the problems of parenthood, you will find, if you have not already, that the world at large is not very understanding of the emotions of parents, that a lot of people have no idea at all about parenthood, and that vast numbers of people thoughtlessly belittle you, even go so far as to undermine your confidence. Some are openly hostile and reject you in your role as parent. On a larger scale you may encounter housing projects or apartment buildings that will not rent to couples with children; there are many restaurants that will do everything in their power to make it clear that they dislike children (from saying so to keeping you waiting endlessly for the least desirable tables). There are recreational facilities and clubs that allow children during certain hours on certain days only. Some of your lifelong friends (without children) may now view you as some kind of oddity, banished from all the other joys of life. If this doesn't tell you that children are in many instances not wanted and that you as a parent are an albatross, I don't know what else will.

It is important for you to know that becoming a parent will change every aspect of your daily life and that it will precipitate many emotional changes as well. More specifically, it will be absolutely impossible for you to come to terms with pregnancy, childbirth, and caring for your baby without understanding that there are going to be problems and difficulties and that you will have to face them. Too many people have a stereotyped picture of parenthood which emphasizes the joys and de-emphasizes the potential problems. For this reason, many people soon find themselves disappointed by parenthood, and some are even overwhelmed. Parenthood is one of the most important, if not the most important, role a human being can take on in life, and yet it is frequently the role people have had the least amount of training for. In particular, they have little or no preparation for the emotional impact of parenthood. Since we human beings purport to place such value on human life, and since our children represent the life of the future, it seems incredible that in our society so little information concerning the responsibilities of parenthood is available.

Until very recently, the socially acceptable response to the confirmation of pregnancy has been depicted unrealistically in films, on the stage, and in our folklore. A husband arrives home from work and greets his wife, "Hi, honey, how was your day?" His spouse, who is sitting on the couch concentrating on her knitting, murmurs, "Hang up your coat, sweetheart, and sit down. I have something to tell you." The startled husband looks intently at his wife and asks, "What is it?" She replies, "I have been to the doctor today, and we are going to have a little visitor." She drops her knitting needles as they rush to embrace. Then they immediately tell each other of their total joy and happiness. Both unequivocally say, "Oh, I'm so happy! Isn't it simply wonderful?"

As you yourself know by now, this scene is clearly fiction. If you compare your emotional reactions when you learned you were going to be a parent with this version, it can only make you wonder if there is something wrong with you. There isn't. It is highly unlikely that your feelings were this simple. At times, you may be overjoyed that you will become a parent, but your reactions will not be all delight and happiness. However it occurred—whether you tried hard to conceive, or whether it came about in an unplanned way, or even if it happened just the way you wanted it to—you should still expect a lot of mixed feelings, and you will soon want answers to an enormous number of questions.

When you really get down to it, very few people have a baby exactly when they want to. Many women find themselves pregnant before they give any deep thought to whether or not they want a child. Fortunately, a lot of people who have been "sitting on the fence" about having a baby find themselves absolutely delighted when the baby is actually born. They are ecstatic with the emotions brought forth by becoming parents. The reality of what they anticipated with mixed feelings becomes a most pleasurable and fulfilling experience. Nevertheless, the reality of pregnancy when it is unexpected can come as quite a shock. If this happened to you, you will find yourself going through many mental contortions to justify your situation, including telling yourself that you really wanted to have a baby at this time anyway. You will probably rationalize the pregnancy by thinking up all kinds of reasons why this is the ideal time to have a baby. By denying that you really didn't want a baby now, you may later end up being overprotective toward your baby in an attempt to compensate for your early ambivalence. Some people take every course available to proclaim their diligence in preparing themselves for parenthood. It has been my experience that when a parent approaches this problem with such disproportionate zeal, he is probably using his in-

tellect to compensate for his emotional ambivalence.

From another point of view, there are couples who try unsuccessfully to conceive for many
years. They look upon each menstrual period as
a milestone of defeat until finally they are vic-
torious and the wife is pregnant at last! When
this situation occurs, it is possible for the child
to suffer. He may be overprotected because parents sometimes overcherish a child who has
been a long time coming. Being disappointed
each month makes a parent highly vulnerable,
and understandably so, to overenthusiasm when
conception finally takes place.

The reason I mention the various ways pregnancy comes about is that in my practice as a
pediatric psychologist I find that this factor con-
tributes heavily to the way parents behave after
the birth of their child. People who do have their
children precisely when they planned to react
differently to their babies than those who didn't
plan at all or those whose plans took many years
to be fulfilled. But whichever way it happened to
you, all of a sudden the role of parent which you
took for granted becomes a stark reality. Of
course, you will experience joy and happiness,
but you can also expect your doubts and misgiv-
ings to cause you great anxiety. Sometimes you
can avoid facing these unpleasant emotions by
saying, "I guess it's natural to feel this way," and
then ignore your feelings so that you do not have
to come to terms with them. But I think this is
unwise. It is much better to recognize your am-

bivalence about becoming a parent so that you can come to terms effectively with both your positive and negative feelings and thereby avoid having your children suffer the consequences of your self-deception. It's only natural to be ambivalent, and parents who accept their natural emotions are best prepared!

Recently I was consulted by the distraught parents of an unhappy three-year-old. They said they wanted to discuss their child's intense separation anxiety and his continuing and increasing infantile behavior. In getting background information, I soon noticed that both parents were quick to lose patience with each other, and I thought they actually seemed more caught up in their own irritability and frustration than they were in their child's unhappiness. Each tended to blame the other for the tense atmosphere at home that each felt was the cause of their child's problem. Every time I attempted to find out more about the three-year-old's problem, the parents would soon revert to discussing their own problems. If I asked for specifics, they would answer in the vaguest terms. I confess I was surprised that they would consult me and then resist getting down to the facts. Intuitively I then asked them, "How did you feel about having your child in the first place?" Actually caught off-guard, they looked at each other in surprise and sputtered, "Well . . . we . . . er . . . of course . . . love our child very much." I said, "That's not what I asked you." And I repeated my question. Immediately the mother became tearful and blurted out, "I have always wanted to say this, but I have always been afraid to. I had such mixed emotions about this child I couldn't stand myself. I always wanted to discuss my feelings with someone, but was afraid that I would be considered an unfit mother. I didn't want anyone to think that I was selfish, and I was afraid my husband would leave me if he realized how I felt when I learned I was pregnant." She went on to describe perfectly normal ambivalence, though she felt incredibly guilty. She described the torture of living with her guilt and admitted that it made her anxious with her child and overprotective. Once the truth was out, she practically diagnosed the child's problem herself. She was able to see how her overprotectiveness caused by her feelings of guilt made the child afraid and caused him to cling to her. She realized quite easily that she was the one who tended to cling to him, and not the other way around. Understandably, the three-year-old reacted as if there were something wrong, which indeed there was —the mother was afraid to leave her child more than he was afraid to leave her. This response to his mother's feelings caused the separation anxiety that the parents came to see me about in the first place. At the end of our session, the father became tearful and said, "If only I had known. Now I see why our feelings changed so much after my wife became pregnant. I never could understand why she seemed so irritated, short-tempered, and impatient with me. If we had known it was normal to feel ambivalence, we would have discussed it openly at that time, and all this trouble could have been avoided."

With the confirmation of pregnancy, some parents-to-be get every book available on child rearing and become completely absorbed in a plenitude of advice and recommendations for raising psychologically healthy children. I cannot tell you how confused this approach can make you. Much of the information available is written not by well-trained professionals but by practicing journalists and self-styled experts who give simple and glib recommendations about parenthood and child rearing. You will also find books written by professionals who provide information in "cookbook style," complete with "recipes" for child rearing. They seldom provide information about the underlying processes of a child's development. Books that are geared to making parenthood easier often neglect information that is essential to your child's emotional and physical well-being. Since they seldom view childhood through a child's eyes, I am always leery of authors who believe that the parent comes first and the child second. It's just not true. To be sure, it is your choice to bring your child into this world in the first place, but after you've done so, it's your responsibility to do all that is best for your child. So, lest you end up totally confused, be selective in what you read and do not try to read everything. If you do, you will only undermine your own confidence. What you ought to do is pick books written by professionals whose extensive experience in working with children and parents helps you understand your child's behavior. You are capable of making intelligent and correct decisions if you know what you should about human behavioral development. Almost all parents want to do what is right for their children. I believe the natural protective tendencies that parents have toward their offspring need to be supported and not undermined by professionals. More than likely, your feelings and instincts are correct. What you need is the self-confidence to follow them.

Days after learning that you are going to have "a little visitor," you will begin to think, "What kind of parent will I be? I am certainly not going to be the way my parents were! I wonder if it's going to be a boy or a girl. Well, I don't care what it is as long as it's happy." As time goes by, you will create a mental image of what your child's gender will be, how she will look, and what your child will be when she grows up. Of course, you want your child to be cute, healthy, brilliant, and happy. You will even find yourself thinking, "I want my child to have all the things I did not have." No matter how much you try to force yourself to empty your mind of these expectations, you will find it extremely difficult, or perhaps even impossible, to do so. There is nothing wrong with this.

In your fantasies, you will find your ideas falling into two categories: one, the image of the parent you expect to be; and two, the image of the child you want. Having these private fantasies is not unnatural, nor is it at all harmful, provided you do not actively work to make them a reality. Nothing undermines a growing child's sense of individuality more quickly than attempts by his parents to mold him to fulfill their own wishes and expectations. Setting up an educational program on your baby's fifth day of life in order that he be accepted twenty years later at Harvard, UCLA, Michigan, or maybe even Cornell, is senseless, and can even be dangerous to your baby's emotional health.

Recently a father and mother made an appointment to consult with me about setting up an educational program for their child. They were apparently deeply concerned and had asked for an early appointment, hopefully the next day. A date was made, but my assistant who arranged it forgot to ask the child's birthday. She just assumed that the child was between four and seven years old. I did too and was very surprised when Mr. and Mrs. Cooper showed up at my office with their eighteen-day-old infant. I innocently asked about the other child they came to consult about and was immediately told they had only one child, Milton. As she reached into her bag for a toy, Mrs. Cooper informed me that Milton was allowed to play only with educational toys. Four times each day he was supposed to spend twenty minutes in programmed play organized by Mrs. Cooper to make sure he followed a sequence of activities geared to his sensory-motor development. I suspected that Mr. Cooper had reservations about this idea but was reluctantly willing to go along with his wife's enthusiastic plans. After all, he thought, she had been a teacher before their marriage and must know what she is doing. As Mrs. Cooper elaborated on the curriculum she had planned so that her child would show reading readiness at an early age, my anxiety began to mount. I watched poor Milton sitting on his father's lap, wanting to be held, caressed, and hugged while Mrs. Cooper jangled her educational toy in front of him. Milton, in his mounting frustration, ignored all her efforts. Mrs. Cooper wanted to know about Milton's indifference to these educational toys and was concerned that his intellectual potential would not be achieved. She really worried, as Mr. Cooper put it jokingly, but with deep sincerity, "that he might not get into my alma mater, the University of Pennsylvania." Of course, I suggested to the Coopers, as I suggest to anyone, that if either parent tends to be overassertive in this way, perhaps the best way to cope with the problem is to have the parents reveal their wishes and fantasies to one another. Each can express feelings openly and frankly, and each can remind the other that wishes and fantasies should not become a plan of action.

I think it is important for you to recognize that you will have two other categories of expectations for your child: those you tell others and those you keep private. Strangely, most parents-to-be deny that these private fantasies exist. The reason for this paradox is that parents unconsciously want their children to fulfill some of their own unfulfilled ambitions. Parents also want their children to experience the same successes and accomplishments they have had in their own lives. In addition, parents wish to treat their children as individuals. They plan to give them, without pressure or coercion, all the freedom necessary to express themselves. This last expectation is usually overtly expressed, but when a parent begins to express his other aspirations for a child, he runs the risk of being accused of acting in an overprotective, overpowering, or coercive manner. Since no one wants to be that kind of parent, any parent has a natural tendency to deny his unconscious wishes and expectations for his child. If you do, don't worry; it's absolutely normal.

As you begin to adjust to your ambivalence about pregnancy—one minute being overjoyed, and the next minute being terrified or depressed—you will find your concentration shifting from your expectations for your child to concern about the discomforts of delivery and the possible complications of childbirth. You are most assuredly not the only one who has these concerns. Many women harbor intense anxiety about the pain of childbirth, the episiotomy that may have to be performed, and the possibility of having the baby so fast that they might not get to the hospital in time. Some of your nervousness undoubtedly stems from experiences you have had and stories you have heard. Some anxiety is instilled by your own parents, by other relatives, and by well-meaning friends, some of whom will be quick to tell you all the details about someone they knew who had a difficult time. Clearly, some anxiety is perfectly normal when you're pregnant. You would have to be incredibly naïve not to know that there is some minor danger in childbirth, but the odds are greatly in favor of things working out well. If you notice carefully what's happening, you will soon find that what other people are doing is increasing your normal anxiety quite unnecessarily. As you progress through your pregnancy, you will probably be surprised at the number of people who will blithely tell you stories that will absolutely scare the daylights out of you. You will hear horror stories about children born with birth defects and deliveries where the complications were frightening. Some people will even encourage you to act as if your pregnancy were an illness and discourage you from engaging in any activity at all. They're wrong. Actually, activity and the motion of the uterus that results provide a growing fetus with healthy amounts of prenatal stimulation. Of course, there may be times during your pregnancy when you feel tired and cannot take your usual routine. At other times, you will find yourself bursting with energy. Either way, act exactly the way you feel like acting and do not let anyone convince you that you are ill. As time goes on, you will hear lots of old wives' tales about determining the gender of your child by the way you are "carrying your baby," or giving it musical talent by attending concerts during your pregnancy, or having it born with a birthmark because you are frightened by some insect. I know one mother whose baby was born with one on his left shoulder in the shape of a mouse. The mother was absolutely convinced that this occurred because she was frightened by a mouse during her pregnancy. Not a single one of these old wives' tales has validity at all, but even if you know this and are not a superstitious person, you may still be amazed at the way you find yourself believing these stories. This reaction is quite common because of the emotional state you find yourself in during pregnancy. The physiological state of being pregnant does affect your emotions, and the awareness of the great responsibility that you are taking on does make you highly sensitive to any information you encounter. The tendency to believe anything you hear will be very great, even if your intellect tells you what you're hearing is clearly nonsense.

Obviously, you will want to minimize the possibilities of things going wrong during pregnancy by arranging for good prenatal care, which will emphasize proper nutrition and include frequent visits to your doctor to check your physical health. But caring for your health will not destroy your worries. You will have to live with them and that will be easier to do if you do not take your fears to be a sign of weakness. Try not to be defensive about them. When you select your obstetrician (which you should do as soon as you learn you are pregnant), do not hesitate to ask all the questions you have concerning your pregnancy and childbirth. Don't hesitate to discuss his beliefs, ideas, and practices as well as his hospital affiliation and the kind of care that the hospital he practices in offers babies and parents. Now is the time to find out such things as whether or not he believes in allowing fathers in the delivery room. It is important that you have the kind of relationship with your obstetrician that enables you to question him freely and to feel confident that he understands your feelings. Make absolutely sure that your doctor is an "askable" person. If you find that his or her advice is contrary to your nature and tends to undermine your confidence, consider finding some other doctor.

The professionals you select for prenatal care and for help during your delivery must have considerable medical skill, but they should also have a sense of humanism, compassion, and respect for your feelings. They should always enhance your understanding and sense of self-importance, and they should never in any way put you down or belittle your questions. There is no reason why you cannot find both technical medical skill and proper consideration for your emotional concerns in the same person. The essential fact of the matter is that you happen to be very important at this particular time. You are going to bring another human being into this world, and you are going to provide the care, love, and protection that will serve to help that child achieve his highest potential both as a productive member of society and as a happy human being.

I am an absolutely firm believer that parenthood means both motherhood and fatherhood. Parenthood is not solely a female responsibility. While bringing up children is an enormous task entailing a lot of hard work and much tedious activity, there are also tremendous pleasures involved. Males as well as females are entitled to the deep satisfactions that come with raising a child and influencing the kind of person he or she will be. Thus, I feel more and more effort should be made to break down the common notion that raising children is a woman's job. Not only do most fathers enjoy being with their children and raising them, but the children themselves gain immeasurably from a father's involvement.

No parent should treat parenthood as a "sometimes job." When a person is a parent, that role should be considered a major responsibility. A significant investment of your time during your child's first five years, followed up by more time through your child's adolescence, will earn you a return on your investment of perhaps fifty or more years of happiness, not only as a parent but as a grandparent too. Fathers ought to devote substantial time to participating in child rearing, and our society ought to help make it possible for them to have that time. I look forward to the day when newspaper and magazine ads as well as television commercials dealing with baby products and child care include a male holding the child, tending to his care, and offering information as an informed parent. I also look forward to the day when courts feel free to consider fathers equal to mothers as custodians of children in divorce cases and not simply assume that the mother will care for the children and the father pay her to do it. It is further my hope that the training of health professionals, including doctors and nurses, will stress the importance of parenthood as well as an understanding of behavioral development and child psychology.

With the confirmation of his wife's pregnancy, the father should begin participating actively in learning the same things that the mother learns about prenatal care and child-rearing practices. It has been my experience that those fathers who do concern themselves with these matters become far more involved in the care of their children than fathers who do not. Moreover, I have observed that fathers who are present when their children are born generally have a far greater sense of the importance of fatherhood than those who are excluded during this dramatic moment. In most instances, sharing this experience improves and strengthens the relationship between husband and wife and transforms it into the kind of relationship that helps mothers become better mothers and fathers better fathers. A few hospitals do encourage fathers to prepare for parenthood and to be present with their wives during childbirth, but I think more effort should be made to increase paternal participation. I feel strongly that fathers should be encouraged to go to classes with mothers during the prenatal period so that they become familiar with the process of labor and delivery, see the labor and delivery rooms in advance, and learn as much as they possibly can about the anticipated experience.

Unfortunately, the traditions of our society tend to exclude fathers. Actually, the exclusion of the male is age-old. The classic movie scene is a good example of what I mean. The woman giving birth is always doing so behind closed doors. Forbidding female figures slip in and out of a thatched hut while various and increasing groans are heard in the background. The father has nothing to do but wait, though occasionally a female stops long enough to instruct the father to boil water or to tear up sheets, without telling him why or what for. As civilization progressed, the father's waiting place was transferred to the hospital hallway outside the delivery room. Nervously, anxiously, he paces back and forth, smoking cigarette after cigarette, doing absolutely nothing. Finally, the nurse informs him that his child has just been born. Then he is charitably allowed a brief glimpse of his child. No wonder he is in a state of near collapse!

Needless to say, excluding the male from the scene of childbirth not only makes it impossible for him to offer comfort and support to his wife during delivery but it makes it impossible for the father to participate emotionally in the event. Worse, his isolation implies rather pointedly that he has no responsibility for child rearing. Since fathers are equally as important as mothers in child rearing, I feel that it is absolutely essential for males to be actively involved. And the best way to get fathers psychologically involved is right from the start, which means at the time pregnancy is confirmed.

-II-

Organizing Your Home for Your Baby

Sooner or later, when you begin to plan for your baby's advent into your home, you are going to be told that you will need help caring for your baby. If you decide you do want help, how you organize that assistance will be important for you, your child, and the relationship between you. Whatever arrangements you eventually make, always remember it's your baby and your responsibility. Actually, most new parents have a strong desire to care for their new baby themselves. Left alone, parents and child soon develop a happy, reciprocal relationship because they both have inborn patterns that make it easy to respond to each other. Any interference with the parents' natural desire to be close to their newborn can interfere with the establishment of the warm and spontaneous relationship between the parents and their baby that is so crucial to the child's healthy development. For this reason, I feel strongly that parents should be the ones who care for their children.

I recommend that when a new baby comes home the assistance that's going to be available should be given to the parents, the mother in particular. Get someone to help with the household rather than with the baby. Then you and your spouse can devote more time to your baby and, if you have them, your other children. Getting someone to assist with the cooking, cleaning, shopping, and other everyday household tasks is far more healthy psychologically for your baby, your other children, and you than allowing someone to take care of your baby. Many parents think hiring an experienced baby nurse is the best thing they can do for their baby. It isn't. Although you may need help, your baby does not. What your baby needs is you. In my opinion, baby nurses generally tend to undermine the confidence of the new parents who hire them. During the critical early months, they keep a baby away from her parents, and they often perpetuate antiquated notions of human behavioral development and antiquated concepts of what a baby is capable of understanding and feeling. Let me give you an example—unusual, to be sure—but one that neatly illustrates exactly what I mean.

Recently, in one of my classes for new parents, a father shared some of the experiences he and his wife had just had with their baby nurse. Apparently, the father's in-laws had paid for the nurse as a present when their grandchild was born. These grandparents had looked hard for a "highly experienced, expensive baby nurse." When they found one, they brought her from some distance to help these new parents for the first two months. As it turned out, this baby nurse, in her attempts to justify her importance as an "experienced baby nurse," totally disregarded the parents' own feelings. In fact, she insisted on following her own ideas, most of which were contrary to the parents' natural inclinations. Soon the mother felt afraid to do anything with her baby without first consulting the nurse for fear that she would do something the nurse would not like. And when the nurse did not approve, the mother was invariably reprimanded —in a smiling way. This mother had the desire to fire the nurse many times, but she felt guilty about the idea because she would seem to be rejecting a present from her parents. Unhappily, the father did not fare any better. He described his enthusiasm and his eagerness to be with his baby when he got home from his office. He would rush into the house and go directly to the baby's room, hoping to pick up the infant and cuddle her. More often than not, he would be met by the baby nurse, in the doorway, smiling and cautioning, "Wait a minute! You have just come in from the cold. You can't pick up the baby. You must wait for your body to warm up so the baby does not catch cold by being chilled." To say the least, the interruption in the father's enthusiasm to get to his little daughter was frustrating and aggravating. Nevertheless, he suppressed his anger, thinking, "If she is as experienced as they say, she must know what's right." As you can see, these poor parents were constantly being thwarted in their attempts to show their feelings toward their new baby spontaneously. Invariably, the nurse intervened, often giving in the process "better advice." The mother, who was nursing her baby, was unable to continue and didn't know why. In describing her breast-feeding experience, she said that every time she fed her baby the nurse would inquire, "Are you positive your daughter is getting enough?" Needless to say, this question, although asked in a pleasant, well-meaning way, eventually caused the mother to doubt whether she was in fact adequate for her child. Her emotional upset soon contributed significantly to her decision to give up breast feeding because it was no longer satisfying. She had been made anxious, and her anxiety soon began to interfere with the free flow of her milk. As it turned out, the nurse's interference was not only psychologically detrimental to the mother, it also contributed to a physiological interruption in the relationship between mother and child. Finally, when two months had gone by, the baby nurse left, to the not-so-secret relief of the parents. Not only, they realized, had this highly experienced, well-meaning nurse shaken their confidence in themselves, but in no way had she helped them cope with their parenthood and their newborn baby's needs. After she left and they were on their own, they had to learn from scratch—just as they would have if the nurse had never been employed. Actually, they were more confused, because they had absorbed some of the idiosyncrasies of the nurse. What little they had learned from her was not only in conflict with their natural tendencies but also in conflict with the kind of parenthood that is in the best interest of any child's healthy emotional development. In retrospect, the parents realized that just having the nurse around made both of them feel that whatever they did was wrong. They also realized that when the grandparents hired the nurse in the first place, they were really, if subconsciously, expressing a lack of confidence in their daughter's ability to be a mother and their son-in-law's ability to be a father.

Another couple recently came to me in despair to discuss some of the problems they were having raising their newborn. They did not have a baby nurse, but they did have the husband's aunt. She had raised three children of her own who were now grown, and she claimed great expertise in raising children. As it turned out, she not only disturbed the normal and natural feelings of these young parents in a way that deprived them of many of the joys of parenthood but she actually went so far as to rearrange their home. For example, the first time Aunt Sheila came to their home, she inspected the room that had been set aside for the new baby. Looking at the parents-to-be in horror, as if they were not only very stupid but totally irresponsible, she exclaimed, "You must move the baby's crib to a different wall immediately! Don't you realize the crib is against an outside wall and that outside walls are cold and damp? You wouldn't want your baby to catch cold and develop pneumonia, would you?" Needless to say, the poor parents were shocked. Without any hesitation they obediently moved the baby's crib. They never dared question Aunt Sheila's remark, though in my opinion there is little or no validity to her concern that the baby would get cold, particularly since these parents lived in a well-insulated house with tight windows. But Aunt Sheila's self-assuredness and the couple's self-effacing response certainly set the tone for their future relationship with the aunt and with their own baby. Aunt Sheila turned out to be a disaster. Finally, with my support, this couple braved family scorn and as tactfully as possible terminated Aunt Sheila's stay in their home.

Some parents who do not want or cannot afford a baby nurse turn to relatives or friends for help after a baby is born. Over the years, this tradition has supposedly enabled mothers to learn child-rearing practices from their own parents and grandparents as well as from friends and other relatives. I myself am not completely sure that this is the best approach to the problem. Much of the advice that new parents get from these same relatives and friends often serves to undermine the confidence of the parents rather than to enhance it. Because these helpers are constantly trying (usually in the most well-meaning way) to coerce the new parent into carrying out their recommendations, they often make the new mother and father feel guilty if their own natural inclinations are contrary to those of the helpful relatives or friends. For example, it is generally the well-meaning helper who tries to convince new parents that their baby should be allowed to "cry it out" because "crying is good for the lungs," or that picking up a crying baby will "only spoil him." They are also quick to point out that a new baby cannot see until she is many weeks old. It almost goes without saying that the proffered knowledge is totally untrue and completely contrary to scientific fact. Nevertheless, these are the kinds of ideas that have been transmitted by relatives and friends who are supposedly trying to help out.

In my many classes with new mothers who have just given birth, I have often noticed that one of their great worries is dealing with their own parents, their in-laws, and other family members. While the new mothers would like to rely upon these people for help, the new parent is afraid to be obligated for fear that it will not be possible to accept help without also accepting advice. Too often their apprehension is justified. Over and over again I have seen situations where new parents have asked grandparents to baby-sit in an emergency. Soon emergency follows emergency, and eventually the grandparents feel free to come and go as they please. When that happens, the new parents, exasperated by their loss of privacy and personal freedom, don't know what to do. They are afraid to tell the grandparents to telephone before they come over or, worse, to tell them to go home so that they can be alone. The parents fear they will offend the grandparents, who might just be thinking, "They call us whenever they need us to baby-sit, but if they don't need us, they don't want us around."

Recently, I had to help one couple extricate themselves from a situation that almost had each of them at each other's throat. The wife's mother traveled 780 miles and moved in for two weeks to help with her new grandson. She was an excellent cook and loved the couple's other child, a three-year-old daughter. The three-year-old had been well prepared for the birth of her brother and initially seemed very happy to have him in the family. However, Grandma assumed that her granddaughter, Nancy, would be jealous and took matters in her own hands. She doted over Nancy, cooking only the foods that Nancy wanted, baked cakes for her, bought her toys, and even had her sleep in her bed to certify her love for Nancy. Whenever Nancy wanted her mother to read to her, or whenever the mother wanted to read to Nancy, Grandma was right on the scene saying, "Oh, don't bother. You take care of the baby. I will read to Nancy so that you can be alone with the baby." While Nancy enjoyed all Grandma's cooking and attention, she began to be apprehensive of the situation—and understandably so. She was becoming estranged from her mother and her baby brother, of whom she seemed initially fond. Grandma, in her attempts to make Nancy feel wanted, actually acted as a wedge between Nancy and the rest of her family. Nancy, understandably, began to wonder why her mother wasn't paying much attention to her and even began to resent her new brother, David. Then Nancy began having nightmares. At night Grandma managed to intercept her as she ran toward her parents' bedroom and took the child to bed with her. She reassured Nancy that everything would be all right and that "Grandma will always love you," in a way that almost implied that her parents wouldn't. Actually, while Nancy was worrying about what was going to happen to her when Grandma left, thinking that she might indeed have been abandoned by her parents, her parents were arguing with each other about Grandma. They were both aware of what Grandma was doing, and while Nancy's father was all for sending Grandma back home, her mother felt she couldn't get herself to send her own mother away. The parents were hardly on speaking terms at that point, which, incidentally, was already two weeks beyond the two weeks Grandma had originally planned to stay. When these parents consulted me, they confessed that they should never have invited Grandma in the first place and said that the longer she stayed the harder it seemed to be to send her home. I helped them set their priorities straight and told them they should show their concern first to their children's feelings, second to their own feelings, and third to Grandma's feelings. They did as I suggested. Grandma left, stating that she didn't feel at all appreciated and that she had been "used." Nevertheless, things got back to normal: Nancy's nightmares ceased, her mother read and played with her, and Nancy began drawing big, colorful pictures to put on David's wall. In short, asking grandparents and other relatives to baby-sit may be a convenience but it may also establish a pattern that allows them to come and go in your home as they please and not as you see fit. If you could sever relations with your relatives whenever you wanted to, there would be no real problem. But often it's impossible because, as we all know, you can't select your parents or your relatives. So if you are going to become involved at all, make sure that you are well fortified—both emotionally and factually. In the end, though, only you can tell whether your parents, relatives, or friends will be inclined to take over or simply help you out when you need it.

If baby nurses are risky and if grandparents and relatives cause problems, where can a mother turn for the help she needs? Perhaps the best place is to her husband. Many people worry about how helpful a father may be after a baby is born simply because he has never shown any great excitement about babies or children. Some women begin pressuring a man until he feels guilty and defensive about his lack of enthusiasm about babies. This is inadvisable, because there are many men whose enthusiasm for babies emerges only after the birth of their own children. When this happens, it not only takes the new mother by surprise but sometimes the father himself, too. "I never thought I would find it as exciting as it is. Seeing my baby grow and being such an important part in that baby's life is simply great," said one father. This kind of statement speaks eloquently for the importance of involving a father in the life of his child.

I am convinced that there is as much of a "fathering instinct" as there is a "mothering instinct," and I believe men are as protective of their children as women, in many instances more so. I speak not only from professional experience with thousands of young parents but on the basis of personal experience as well. Raising my own children, spending a great deal of time with them and helping them learn about trusting relationships is terribly rewarding. Watching them satisfy their curiosity while they gain skills for dealing with the normal encounters of everyday life still provides me with one of the greatest satisfactions in my own life. I believe nothing can give a person a greater sense of self-esteem than having children who are trusting, happy, curious, and capable of coping. For any father, having a child really should be more than having a "chip off the old block," or adding a "junior" to his own name. Fatherhood does involve hard work, great responsibility, considerable amounts of time, but it also provides untold quantities of joy, satisfaction, and happiness. Only by eliminating the sex-role stereotypes about child rearing can we free fathers to feel more significant in the lives of their newborn babies.

I feel strongly that what has in the past been called home economics should now be revised and renamed "human survival training." As I recall, in first grade, our teacher taught us that the basic necessities of life were food, clothing, and shelter. Furthermore, she pointed out that care of the offspring was an important element in the survival of many species. I have never forgotten those remarks and their implications. It is true that within a family structure there has to be some separation of responsibility. How the separations are made depends upon cultural background, life-style, and the personal feelings of each family member. I believe it important that these responsibilities be assigned in such a way that the personal exploitation of any individual family member does not result from an arbitrary breakdown of whose job it is to do what. Nevertheless, I would like to see our educational system make the concept of "human survival training" available to all children, both boys and girls. Human survival training would involve learning the basic elements of preparing food and the basics of nutrition. In addition, it would include training in the basic concepts of clothing the body for protection as well as the care and maintenance of that clothing. Providing shelter clearly involves understanding the structure of a house and its maintenance, including cleaning and electrical and plumbing repairs. It also involves such things as painting, carpentry, washing windows, and vacuuming. Human survival training as I envision it would not be complete without teaching a basic knowledge of healthy child development, and the role and responsibilities of parenthood. This kind of human survival training would have no sex-role implications, the way home economics, which is offered almost solely to young women, now does.

Once human survival training is common in our schools and in our society it would have numerous benefits. Even if a family decided to designate various routine responsibilities to certain family members—cooking for the female, perhaps, shopping for the male, housecleaning for both, or whatever fits the individual family's particular choices—the fact that all the adult members of that family had received the same human survival training would enable each to take over the responsibilities of the other if the need arose. If the woman in the household preferred, in the old tradition, to handle the cooking, shopping, housecleaning, and not be involved in earning money, she would still have the benefit of adequate understanding and cooperation from the rest of the family, her husband in particular. By the same token, if human survival training taught a man about child rearing as well as home maintenance and food preparation, he could then easily take on these responsibilities if he and his wife decided that the wife should be the primary earner of family funds.

By giving all members of the family skills in more aspects of family life, human survival training can only strengthen the existence of the family unit. Since I believe in the family as the best milieu for raising children, human survival training can enable us to have happier, healthier children. In addition, if children grow up in the kind of family environment I have in mind, they will have the opportunity to identify with parents who can move freely among all the assignments whose completion is necessary for the maintenance of healthy family life. The children in the family will not associate any one role with either masculinity or femininity. I consider that to be an ideal arrangement for parents and their children.

-III-

Whether to Breast Feed or Bottle Feed

The decision whether to breast feed or bottle feed should be given ample consideration well before your baby is born. Unfortunately, too many parents wait until the last moment. Sometimes a mother who is undecided is asked in the delivery room itself to make up her mind whether or not she plans to breast feed. The obstetrician wants her decision so he or she will know whether or not to inject a hormone that will interfere with the production of the mother's milk. The doctor does want to know what you plan to do, but this is hardly the right moment for you to decide. So don't wait until the last minute and, more important, don't make the decision without giving careful consideration to all the ramifications.

In my experience, mothers who are considering breast feeding have two major concerns: First, "Will my baby be able to get enough milk from me? Will I be able to produce enough to satisfy her needs?" Second, mothers wonder, "Will I be tied down if I breast feed my child?" In response, I usually say that there is no reason to assume that a mother will not produce enough milk to satisfy her baby's needs; and that while breast feeding obviously requires the mother's presence, it does not tie her down any more than is in the best interests of her child.

Unfortunately, there is a great deal of misinformation given about the choice between breast feeding and bottle feeding. Worse yet, many doctors or other health professionals when asked their advice transmit their own prejudices in a manner that may undermine a mother's natural inclination one way or another. Recently, in one of my classes, I encountered a mother who described in detail her frustration at having made the decision not to breast feed her first child. She realized she had made a mistake, and she was angry with her doctor for having said, "Why do you want to bother? You don't really want to be tied down to your baby forever, do you?" The image the doctor created in this mother's mind at that moment was one of breast feeding as a burdensome activity. Obviously, immediately following her delivery, she felt she needed no further burdens, so she made her choice not to breast feed. Her later frustration was intensified because she had let herself be influenced.

Clearly, there are subtleties in the way people provide you with factual information, and at times these subtleties could determine your choice. Your key defense against this involves self-awareness and a determination to gather as many facts as you can—facts, not opinions.

All things being equal, I am inclined to recommend breast feeding, though I do not take a hard and fast position on this matter. I seldom encounter a mother who chose to breast feed and later regretted it. On the other hand, I have spoken with many mothers who regretted having made the decision to bottle feed. Some women do feel very strongly that they do not wish to breast feed, and I would not pressure them. But I confess I would be inclined to tell any reluctant mother enough about breast feeding so that the facts might counteract any prejudices she happened to have. Then I'd accept her choice. However, if a mother is generally undecided, I would probably urge her to breast feed because in general breast feeding is not a problem. The plain fact is that most women do achieve a satisfactory breast feeding relationship with an infant.

I am inclined to feel that in the course of evolution and through the process of natural selection, the milk provided by a human mother is more geared to her baby than the milk of another species. Many noted nutritionists state that the proportion of solid to liquid in mothers' milk is better geared to the physiology of a baby than cows' milk. Generally speaking, babies develop an allergy less frequently to their own mothers' milk than to formula. Breast-fed babies do not have a sour smell when they spit up their milk, but bottle-fed babies do. In short, it seems as if nature provided the right balance in human milk for human babies. Incidentally, another argument in favor of breast feeding is that the shape of a mother's breast prevents her baby from becoming a tongue thruster. Tongue thrusting sometimes leads to a lisp or creates pressure against the teeth that may cause dental malformations. The rubber nipples used on bottles are sometimes shaped in a way that does not prevent tongue thrusting. It is, therefore, no surprise that people in the speech-therapy field notice fewer lisps among children who were breast fed. Best of all, many mothers who breast feed tell me they find it very convenient to have a supply of milk available at all times, warmed to the right temperature, and ready to serve.

Unfortunately, many women who hold breast feeding in high esteem set it up as a challenge. Any difficulty a person might have in effective breast feeding is interpreted by these people as a personal failure. For example, as I spoke recently to a group of new mothers in the hospital, one mother battered away at me with one question after another concerning the importance of breast feeding to a baby's emotional health. This mother's manner of questioning me as well as her anguished attempt to hold back the tears welling up in her eyes told me she was very anxious. When I mentioned that she seemed upset, she immediately confessed that her baby was sluggish and didn't show a strong desire to suck at her nipples. She broke into tears as she said, "All my friends were successful in breast feeding their children. I'm a failure. My baby wants the bottle from the nurse more than me. I was determined to make this work, and I failed horribly." The fact of the matter was that she received a lot of sedation during her labor which made her baby sluggish. But this sluggishness, which was not this mother's fault, had made her ashamed to face her friends, because, as she saw it, "They succeeded and I failed."

The tension and anxiety that accompanies this approach to breast feeding is not in the best interest of a warm, gratifying parent-child relationship. Moreover, emotional tension itself can interfere with effective breast feeding because the "let-down reflex," the mechanism that allows milk to flow freely from the mother's breast to the infant, is markedly affected by tension. Obviously, any mother who views breast feeding as a challenge is tense. Her tension interferes with the let-down reflex which in turn decreases the supply of milk, and this often leads to a feeling of failure, which then increases the challenge, then the tension, and finally the feeling of failure. This cycle is not only uncomfortable and upsetting to a mother but, more important, it destroys the potentially warm and gratifying mother-infant relationship that usually flowers when a baby is breast-fed.

As I have said, there is a substantial interplay between the psychological and the physiological elements that enter into the breast-feeding relationship. In the old days, mothers used to be encouraged to drink beer when they were breast feeding. The supposition was that beer increased the production of milk. Actually, it was not the beer itself, but the effects of the beer on the mother that increased the flow of milk. The alcohol in the beer tended to relax the mother. When she relaxed, the let-down reflex facilitated the milk flow. The point I am making is not supposed to benefit the beer-producers' association but to emphasize the importance of a mother's attitude in successful breast feeding.

Sometimes it is not possible for a mother to continue breast feeding, even though she tried initially. There may be some unexplained reason why she did not succeed, or perhaps she developed an infection (which is not an altogether good reason for discontinuing breast feeding), or maybe her nipples cracked and the resulting pain and discomfort forced her to discontinue. It can be very discouraging when something like this occurs, but if you approach breast feeding in a flexible and open-minded way to begin with, you should not feel a loss of self-esteem or regard yourself as a failure if bottle feeding necessarily becomes the way you feed your baby.

Whether you are planning to breast feed or bottle feed, you should understand something about your baby's emotional needs as they exist right after birth. A baby has a strong need for sucking satisfaction. He is born with this reflex, and it must be gratified if he is to be first a happy, satisfied infant and later a stable adult. Studies have shown that frustration of this early infantile need can lead to adult behavior patterns that are attempts to find gratification for these early frustrated needs in some indirect way. Examples include excessive smoking, immoderate use of alcoholic beverages, and sometimes an insatiable desire to consume food. Strange as it may seem, a newborn baby has no real concept of eating. When her stomach is empty and needs food, the baby will get hunger pangs which are actually minor stomach contractions. Because these contractions will be moderately discomforting, they will generally cause a baby to fret or cry. When this occurs, any baby's need to suck increases because sucking is a baby's primitive way of coping with discomfort. When her mother begins to feed the baby, the sucking need begins to be satisfied. At first, the gratification that a baby obtains while feeding is primarily associated with satisfying her sucking needs. The amount of food consumed is secondary. Breast feeding, being nature's way, is an excellent system for simultaneously satisfying both the sucking need and the need for food. Breast-fed babies get most of their milk in the first few minutes of sucking. This assures that the baby gets the proper amount of nutrient before the sucking need can possibly be satisfied. Then the baby continues sucking on the breast not because the baby is hungry but to obtain sufficient sucking satisfaction so she can relax and go to sleep. When the sucking need is satisfied, and not before, the baby releases her mother's breast, relaxes, and goes to sleep.

Contrast this efficient system with the bottle-fed baby, who gets his milk supply at the same rate during the entire feeding. Parents who bottle feed their babies sometimes find that their babies have enormous appetites. After consuming one bottle, the infant devours a second and may still want more. In my opinion, it is highly unlikely that the baby actually needs that much food. It is more likely that he may have to consume that amount of food to satisfy his sucking needs completely. If you notice that your baby seems to be acting this way, get some nipples with small holes so that your baby has to suck a little harder to get his food. In this way, he can gratify his sucking needs without consuming an inordinate amount of milk. Incidentally, I have noticed that the holes in the nipples provided with commercially prepared formulas are usually large. This benefits the company that makes the formula, not your baby. And while your baby consumes quantities of unnecessary formula, the manufacturer happily reports greater sales. He also advertises that babies fed on his formula gain weight faster than breast-fed babies.

Whatever method you select for feeding your newborn, it is essential that your baby gain his or her sucking satisfaction in conjunction with the feeding process. A baby who achieves her sucking gratification while she eats is less inclined to show a need for continued sucking at other times. Generally, she will show less tendency to become a thumb-sucker and will usually stop putting objects in her mouth at an earlier age than babies whose sucking needs have been thwarted at feeding time. Many years ago, Dr. David Levy conducted a study in which he conclusively demonstrated that puppy dogs who were weaned before they were psychologically ready tended to be destructive with their mouths well into adulthood. These dogs chewed up chair and table legs, tore bedspreads and ripped curtains throughout their lives. However, those dogs whose sucking needs were gratified as part of the feeding process until they were psychologically ready to give it up showed no sign of these traits. Significantly, experimenters attempting to modify the behavior of the destructive dogs found it very difficult, if not impossible, to reverse the tendencies established in early life.

I think it is important for your baby to gain a sensation of something going into his stomach while his sucking need is being gratified. In this way, the child soon learns to associate sucking gratification with the feeding process. If sucking satisfaction is functionally separated from feeding, say when a child is constantly allowed to use a pacifier, sucking can become a habit pattern which is no longer related to its original purpose, namely, to cause a baby to eat. Since a child's need for sucking satisfaction normally diminishes with age, he will eventually give it up spontaneously if he is not coerced too early, if he is not under emotional stress, and if he has not begun to associate sucking satisfaction with some physical object other than food.

In addition to the sucking need, a newborn baby has a distinct need for parental contact. Your baby requires fondling, stroking, warmth, touching, and the sound of your voice as well as the image of your face. Happily, your baby's need to eat forces the kind of close physical contact that tends to meet your baby's need for closeness. In a way, feeding a child forces the kind of mother-infant contact that is essential for healthy emotional development. Breast feeding, particularly. It is not possible, as it is with a bottle, to prop up your breast, go into the next room, and read a book—at least I hope it is not possible! Because of your infant's need for parental contact, if you decide to bottle feed, I particularly urge you to hold your baby during feedings. Along the same lines, it is not a bad idea for a mother to hold her baby against her bare body while bottle feeding so that her baby can get the full experience of touch, taste, and smell that helps establish the identity of his mother. Close contact during the feeding experience is most gratifying to a baby.

Lest I sound too enthusiastic about breast feeding, let me say I am inclined to recommend giving a baby an occasional bottle even if you decide to breast feed, partly to accustom your child to this form of feeding if his mother's absence makes it necessary and partly to give the father an opportunity to feed his baby. By the way, if you to decide to get your baby accustomed to an occasional bottle right from the beginning, make sure that the mother gives this occasional bottle until your baby becomes used to it. If the baby, right from the start, associates breast feeding with her mother and bottle feeding with others, your baby may well begin to associate a bottle with separation from her mother. If the mother first introduces the occasional bottle and later the father gives this bottle while mother is present, eventually the baby will not associate the bottle with maternal separation. I know that many people who are ardent proponents of breast feeding take a strong position against even an occasional bottle. They object because they think that an occasional bottle will weaken the breast-feeding relationship, or because they feel that mothers' milk is nutritionally most beneficial to a child. I don't find these arguments to be very convincing. But even if they were, I still feel that flexibility and the other advantages of an occasional bottle far outweigh the disadvantages. Moreover, treating breast feeding as an all or nothing affair tends to discourage some people from starting to breast feed in the first place.

When do you stop breast feeding? This question really has no clear answer. While some supporters of breast feeding encourage parents to continue to breast feed a baby for as long as three years, I am inclined to feel that breast feeding beyond two years tends to increase a baby's dependency on its mother, just at the time when he is showing, and you should be encouraging, a greater sense of independence. When babies are breast-fed after they are two years old, I am forced to question whether it's done for the good of the baby or for the mother's own satisfaction. I don't mean to imply that in all cases continued breast feeding is unwise, but I do think one can fairly question the need for continued breast feeding as a way of analyzing the psychology of the child's feeding experience. However, when you stop breast feeding, don't force your baby to give up the satisfaction that accompanies his sucking. If your baby still needs sucking gratification after you wean him from the breast, use a bottle until his sucking need has been outgrown.

The question of breast feeding versus bottle feeding is one that parents should face themselves, particularly taking into consideration the feelings of the mother, since breast feeding would naturally concern her the most. Be aware that many of your friends and relatives, perhaps even your doctor, will try to influence you, often in response to their own feelings rather than out of consideration for your own desires. Get whatever facts you can, give it careful thought, and do not lose sight of your own wishes. If you feel strongly against breast feeding, don't force yourself to try it. On the other hand, if you are undecided about breast feeding, I would urge you to attempt it. Breast feeding works so well for most mothers, perhaps because nature intended that it should. It particularly strengthens the relationship between parent and infant—and that is the most important thing about feeding your child. You must enjoy it and so must she. Basically, that's really more important to her sound psychological development than the source of supply.

-IV-

Preparing Your Older Child for the New Baby

Most parents who have a child and are expecting another are acutely aware of the problems created by sibling rivalry. They sense that inept parental handling can lead to intense jealousy, severe regression, or serious rebellion on the part of the older child. One of the questions I am most frequently asked is how parents can avoid sibling rivalry. Recently, I was consulted about sibling rivalry by a mother who was due to have her baby in a month. She had a two-and-a-half-year-old at home with whom she had spent a great deal of time. This mother had read many books about child rearing, knew about sibling rivalry, and acknowledged her older child's need for individual attention after her baby would be born. The purpose of her consultation with me was to find out what she could do to minimize her older child's jealousy of the new baby since she was somewhat anxious that her older child would resent the baby. This mother had already discussed her problem with her pediatrician. Among other things, she had advised her to go to the local toy store, buy a few dozen inexpensive toys, and individually wrap each of them. The pediatrician told this mother to give one of these toys to her older child each time a visitor brought a gift for the new baby. The pediatrician said this procedure would minimize the older child's jealousy and prevent him from feeling left out. The mother thought this idea seemed reasonable. In fact, she had heard other people recommend it.

I told this mother that I disagreed with this method of handling sibling rivalry because it can have just the opposite effect of what the parents want. I believe if you give your older child a little something each time your baby gets a gift, you only teach your older child to expect that he will get a present every time your baby gets one. An older child dealt with in this manner quickly learns to inspect what he got and what the baby got to see which is better. And believe me, your older child is sure to find inequities at the most minute level. He will locate scratches and blemishes barely visible to the naked eye. In short, the method recommended by the pediatrician places too much emphasis on material things, does not face up to the child's concern about the extent of your love, and is not realistic. I explained to the mother who consulted me that it would be better to tell her older child that people who visit babies often bring presents and that many people who visited him when he was a baby brought him presents. Then she should go on to say that because her older child is not a baby, he will not be treated like a baby, but will be treated differently.

I can assure you that your older child's real interest is not in presents, but in being important, in being assured that he is still loved, and in receiving some undivided time and attention from you. No toy or other object can ever satisfy these needs in your older child. You absolutely have to convey the feeling that your child is still important to you through your actions. You must give your older child your full attention without his having to demand it, or worse, to engage in destructive or hostile behavior in order to get your interest. Any child who is given attention only as a result of aggressive or destructive behavior will soon learn to rely upon it as the method for gaining attention. If you begin by trying to equalize everything between your older child and your baby, you will find it hard to get across the concept that individuals are different and are treated differently. Later you will have trouble handling matters such as different bedtimes, different school hours, and different family responsibilities. If your child recognizes from the start that your love for each of your children is different because each of them is different, especially different in age, then you will be free to treat them differently. It's much easier in the long run than constantly trying to promote equality.

One of the best ways to avoid sibling rivalry is to begin preparing your child for the new baby shortly after your pregnancy is confirmed. Your pregnancy is indeed an exciting event that will soon evoke the kind of curiosity and fascination that children have about human existence and life in general. It is perfectly natural for your older child to want to learn how a life begins, how a baby grows, and how it gets born. I see no reason whatsoever not to satisfy your child's curiosity about these matters, since she is sure to have many questions. She will want to know, among other things, just how the baby comes out. It is important for children to know exactly how a baby leaves its mother's body. Many well-meaning parents confuse their children on this point by directly misinforming them. They explain that, "The baby comes out the bellybutton," or "the bottom." Other parents avoid the subject entirely and leave their child to his own imagination. This is wrong. A child should be specifically told that the baby is growing in the mother's uterus, that it started as an egg (or a cell) that came from a place called the ovary and was fertilized by something like a seed, called a sperm, from the father. Nine months later, when the baby is full grown and ready to be born, the vagina gets bigger so that the baby can come out. A doctor usually helps the baby come out, and then the vagina gets smaller again. This description not only provides accurate information (except in cases where Cesarean section is performed) but it also helps children understand the female anatomy. And children will find nothing traumatic about this explanation nor anything disgusting about it. Eventually you will be able to make it clear that when the baby is ready to be born, you will have to go to the hospital for a few days so that your doctor can help the baby get born. Explain that after a baby is born, the mother needs to rest in the hospital for a while, and doctors and nurses have to watch over the baby carefully for a few days to make sure that he is completely healthy. Your child will then be prepared for the separation that takes place at the time of the baby's birth. Since that separation will be one of his greatest concerns, be sure to say that you will miss your older child while you are in the hospital and will be unhappy being away from him.

Your child will have many questions to ask concerning what the hospital is like and what happens there. Answer your child's questions honestly in a way that he can understand. If you are not sufficiently familiar with hospitals to answer his questions, tell your child that you do not know but will try to find out.

When you are discussing your pregnancy, your hospital stay, and the coming of a sibling with your child, you should encourage an atmosphere of complete openness and honesty. This will make it easier for your child to tell you about her feelings about this change in the family. It often helps to ask your child how she feels about having another brother or sister, and you ought to know that it is perfectly normal and natural for an older child to have certain feelings of ambivalence about, possibly even to dislike, the idea of having a baby in the family. The quality and intensity of the child's feelings will vary according to many factors—the age interval between the child and the baby, the amount of time you spend with your children, the degree of patience and understanding you have toward your children, and certainly, the way in which you have prepared your child for the advent of his or her sibling.

If your child is unenthusiastic, explain that negative feelings are by no means wrong, but then get across to your child that although he does not have to like the new baby, he absolutely cannot hurt him. It is far healthier for everyone involved if both the feelings of love and the feelings of hostility can be discussed rather than suppressed, but, obviously, physical expressions of hostility are not going to be tolerated. Actually, I am inclined to believe that if a child expresses an unconditional desire for a new brother or sister, he may be conforming to his parents' expectations and not revealing his real feelings. After all, why shouldn't a child be apprehensive and ambivalent about a sibling? A new brother or sister is going to change the family constellation, maybe for the worse. And a child invariably wonders, "Will they still love me after the baby is born and comes home?"

Telling your child that you are going to have a baby well in advance of the baby's birth should give you ample time to certify your love and help your child cope with his ambivalence.

The principle of honest preparation applies to children of all ages, though it is difficult to put into practice if the older sibling is under the age of three. Children between approximately eighteen months and three years have difficulty conceptualizing; their emotional expressions are crude; they are normally negativistic and defiant; they still need a great deal of their parents' time to help them come to terms with their infantile needs, such as weaning and toilet training; and they have not established a real sense of independence. All these factors make them particularly vulnerable to feeling in some way compromised by the birth of a sibling. A child under the age of three, no matter what he has been told in advance, often reacts negatively to a new baby, and his reaction puts tremendous stress on his parents. Invariably, they feel that, "There must be something wrong with our older child, or she would not be so defiant and rebellious." While I understand what makes a parent feel this way, I do not agree with the conclusion, despite the opinions of many of my colleagues who are inclined to attribute the negativism and the defiance of the child to sibling rivalry. I think they have cause and effect mixed up. Any child this age is normally negative and defiant, whether or not there's a baby in the family. If there does happen to be a baby, then the older child easily picks that to be negative and defiant about. However, having children three or more years apart in age does help diminish later sibling rivalry, to say nothing of easing the demands made on parents. If a child is three or older, she is ready for nursery school or some other kind of organized educational group. She is also capable of establishing some life of her own and having friends outside the home. She is capable of understanding the fascination of the reproductive process. Best of all, her ability to exist independently of you makes it easier for you to give each child a certain degree of undivided time and attention.

Everyone, and not only parents, should understand what a new sibling means to an older child. Sooner or later we all visit the homes of parents who have just had a new baby. The visitor invariably wonders whether he should bring a present not only for the new baby but for the older child as well. The visitor also plans what to say to the older child. Naturally, most adults are happy and delighted, even ecstatic, about the birth of a relative's or friend's new baby. Often they expect the other children in the family to feel the same way. So they approach the situation in an intellectual manner without really considering the older child's emotions. They tend to "push" love, expecting the older sibling of the newborn baby to acquiesce in their approach: "Don't you just adore your new brother? Isn't he cute? Oh, you're so lucky to have such a fine little baby." The well-meaning adult who makes these remarks wants to make the older child love the new baby. Unfortunately, this approach is exactly wrong, not because the person who adopts it is ill-willed but because it lacks a general understanding of what is going on in the child's mind. Too many adults have, it seems, forgotten what it is like being a child.

I have spoken to innumerable new mothers, new fathers, and siblings of new babies and have come to realize how little general understanding there is about the feelings of siblings. I remember one mother, well-educated with a degree in child development, proudly telling me two days after the birth of her second child exactly what she had said to her two-and-a-half-year-old. To prepare him for being alone while she went to the hospital to deliver, she had explained she was departing on a week's vacation. That was her entire explanation. When I asked why she selected this approach, she said, "I wanted to avoid making it a traumatic event for my child." Simple common sense will tell you how short-sighted this well-meaning woman was. First of all, she told a lie simply to put off telling the truth. Second, she set up the situation to be far more "traumatic" than it might have been. Third, the way she dealt with the situation made it impossible for her to help her child cope with his problem. Needless to say, coming home with a newborn baby after a supposed week's vacation proves that a parent has not told the truth. It can lead to distrust of the parent, not to mention serious apprehension about the parent's vacationing in the future. At the same time, covering up the situation in this way or any other communicates the idea that having a new brother or sister is so serious a matter that parents can't be open, direct, and honest about it.

I recall another situation where a mother, having explained all about her pregnancy some months before, telephoned her older child from the hospital right after the baby was born. "Your new sister is so cute," said this mother. "I told her all about you, and she can't wait to meet you. She loves you so much already that she even has a present to give you when she sees you." Imagine the reaction of her two-and-a-half-year-old. He had been told about the baby growing in his mother's uterus, and he had been told that when the baby was ready to be born, his mother would have to go to the hospital to have the doctor help the baby get born. In his curious, young mind, he could not help but wonder, "Where did that little kid get a toy for me? Does my mother have some kind of toy store in her uterus? How can that baby love me or even like me? It doesn't even know me. If it likes me, how am I supposed to feel about it when I don't even know it. I think I might not like it, but my mother will sure be angry with me if I don't love it and it loves me." As you can see, this two-and-a-half-year-old has been unnecessarily loaded with an incredible burden. His mother's approach only set the stage for confusion, significant ambivalence, and an unfair expectation that the older child love his new sister. His mother put him in a position which could only increase his resentment toward both his new sister and his mother. It might even have lead him to feel intensely guilty for not being able to live up to his parents' expressed expectations.

You must remember that the birth of a sibling causes a child to question whether or not he was good enough for his parents. Any child inevitably wonders, "If they were really happy with me, why did they have to go off and have another child?" In this example, no one is helping the child cope with his concern that his parents might not love him. On the contrary, they are all trying to cover up the problem or put the burden of solving it on him. This approach is not only unfair, but ineffective. It can only lead to the opposite of what the parents are trying to accomplish.

Sometimes parents in their anxiety to avoid sibling rivalry overreact. One young couple, in their exuberant attempt to make their two-and-a-half-year-old feel more important and involved, told their child, "The only reason we had the new baby was for you. We wanted you to have a little sister of your own because we wanted you to have someone to play with. You see, we love you so much, even more than the baby." Not only are these statements untrue but they place the full responsibility for the baby's existence on the older child. To begin with, the child probably doesn't believe what she's been told, and as a result, she will be less inclined to trust her parents. Then, as she sees her parents being affectionate toward her little sister, she will be convinced that they love the baby more than they love her, whether they do or not. In addition, this approach begs the question of the equality of parental love and will make the child more aware than ever of the inevitable differences in the way her parents express their feelings and the frequency with which they do so.

In the case of these exuberant parents, three weeks after the baby was born, the two-and-a-half-year-old, crying bitterly, exclaimed, "Take the baby back to the hospital, I don't want her! She is no good and no fun to play with. I didn't want her! Take her back, take her back, take her back!!!" Her parents were hard put to deal with this outburst, since they had set the stage for it themselves. From the child's point of view, why shouldn't her parents take the baby back? After all, they had had the baby only for her, so why should she be forced to keep her? Actually, it is quite common for young children even when properly prepared for the birth of a sibling to ask that the new baby be taken back to the hospital. In fact, children often say, "Let's put the baby in the garbage. I don't want him anymore." If this particular suggestion is made in your home, it does not mean you have a psychopath on your hands. It is simply a logical expression of a young child's resentment toward a new baby. After all, what does he see you do with things you don't want? You put them in the garbage! You really need not be alarmed when a young child makes remarks like this.

One of the most overlooked ways to minimize sibling rivalry is to introduce your older child to your newborn baby immediately. Ideally, you should take your older child to the hospital to visit his mother and the new baby as soon as possible. Once the visit takes place, the older child readily becomes a part of the total event. Seeing the new baby and seeing his mother in good health, if perhaps a little fatigued, allows your child to know what's happened. He will no longer have to live with whatever fantasies he had about what his mother went through to give birth to a baby. Many little children get the idea that the moment a baby is born, the baby will right away want to come home and play. Seeing the baby in the hospital conveys immediately that the baby is so tiny that he is not really capable of playing. Along the same lines, a four-and-a-half-year-old whose mother had just given birth to his sister—and was still in the hospital—drew two pictures for me. One drawing was of three people—the baby, the mother, and himself. It was fascinating: In his picture the mother was about three-fourths of the length of the paper, the new baby was the full length of the paper, and he was only one-third of the length of the paper. Clearly, he felt that the baby was more important to his mother than he was, so much so that the baby was bigger than his mother and three times his size. My interpretation of his feelings was confirmed in his next drawing, which was a picture of the new baby and his mother in bed together, snuggling with each other. The baby was almost as big as his mother, who was drawn with her body cut open at the abdomen, dripping with blood. Not only were the mother and the baby showing great love to each other, but the child saw the birth of his sibling as a mutilation of his mother. In discussing this picture with little David, he told me that they were "loving each other." I asked what they were thinking, and he said, "Only of each other—no one else." He explained further that his mother was "all opened up and bleeding from where the doctor took the baby out." I arranged to have David visit his mother in the hospital and also see the new baby. David seemed initially taken aback as he looked his mother over from head to toe while she stood before him with open arms ready to embrace him. He said, "But, but, you're . . . all right, you're not opened up." As she held him, he looked around and said, "It's beautiful here. What nice flowers! Where are the doctor's instruments?" Apparently he expected to find what he had depicted in his drawings, plus the doctor's surgical instruments. When David's mother took him to see his new sister, David, wide-eyed, commented, "She's . . . she's . . . so little. I thought she'd be—" He never finished that sentence, but its meaning was in his drawing.

I have observed a number of very young children who came to visit the same day their mothers gave birth. Not once did I observe anything that was psychologically upsetting to the child. In fact, I remarked upon the opposite. The little children were delighted to see their mothers, and the mothers took great pleasure in showing the new babies to their older children. Needless to say, the visits precipitated many questions about the newborn babies that made the actual homecoming a casual event. Since sibling visitation is important to your child's emotional health, I sincerely hope that hospitals will modify the antiquated procedures which now keep little children away from the maternity wards. Antiseptic conditions, in whose name present procedures are invoked, can, I believe, be assured in other ways, so that siblings can have the psychological advantages of visiting their mothers and the new babies. It always seems highly unfair to me that of all the family members, it should be the little siblings that find it hardest to participate in this great family event. Imagine how they must feel hearing aunts, uncles, grandparents, and friends commenting on the new baby whom they have not yet had a chance to see.

Some proponents of the idea that children should not be allowed to come to hospitals to visit their mothers or the new babies point out that having the older child visit causes a series of separations rather than a single separation for the four- or five-day period of the usual confinement. They feel the increased number of separations is harmful. I do not agree. If the child happens to be reluctant to leave his mother after a visit and cries, this is unfortunate but not emotionally disastrous. It is far worse for any child to experience one prolonged separation than a series of short ones. Of course, reassuring your child between each of the short separations that he is still part of the now-enlarged family helps a lot.

It is a fact of life, including childbirth, that things do not always turn out the way we expect. Sometimes they go wrong in rather insignificant and minor ways, but sometimes the departure from what we anticipate is serious, perhaps even tragic. While this is not usually the case in childbirth, it does happen. Unfortunately, some babies are born with defects or deformities, and some are stillborn. There are also miscarriages. So I think you should understand the psychological implications of these events and know how to help your older child cope with his feelings if these unfortunate circumstances should occur. In any case, these matters are sure to arise and be asked about, even if your children simply hear words like "stillborn," "premature baby," "Cesarean section," "incubator," and "miscarriage" used, perhaps in a discussion of someone else's misfortune.

If you have properly prepared your child and explained that it takes nine months for a baby to grow before she is ready to be born, your explanation will have implied that the baby will be born alive without birth defects and that she will not require any special care. You need not explicitly explain in advance that something may go wrong. To do so just heightens your child's anxiety and provokes questions that are not really appropriate. If a miscarriage then occurs, tell your child that the baby began to grow, but something went wrong and it stopped growing. Perhaps you can say that it's like planting seeds in a garden; some of them grow and others do not. Be sure you emphasize that nothing your child felt, wished, or did caused the miscarriage and that it was one of those things that absolutely no one could prevent. Likewise, if the baby is stillborn, your explanation should be along the same lines: "The baby began growing and something went wrong so that the baby did not grow right and could not be born alive." You can explain a deformity in a baby in much the same way. Again emphasize that nothing your child felt, wished, or did caused this to happen, and that no one, not even doctors, nurses, or anyone else, could have done anything about it. If a baby is born prematurely, the best explanation is that the child was born before he or she was completely ready to be born and is not strong enough or big enough to come home right away. This statement satisfactorily explains why the child is being taken care of in a premature nursery, usually in an incubator.

The reason you have to handle all these unexpected situations directly, openly, and honestly is to prevent an older child from getting confused ideas or developing feelings of guilt. Young children do go through a phase in psychological development where they believe that events can occur magically. Since most older siblings have mixed feelings about the arrival of a new brother or sister, they may at times have wished that the baby would not be born. If in fact something happens so that the baby is not born, your child may feel guilty. He may even worry that his wishes magically came true. A miscarriage or stillbirth is precisely the kind of situation that causes a child to feel this way. To destroy this misconception you have only to tell your child what did in fact occur. Give an accurate explanation at the time so that you will not later have to correct a misconception the child created for himself. Little children need explanations, and if explanations are not provided, they make them up in their own minds.

Sometimes a child's misconceptions do not become immediately evident. A parent may not even realize that his child has a confused concept. For example, I recall one situation where a mother began to miscarry. She and her husband and their three-year-old all rushed to the hospital. As soon as they arrived, the mother was put into a wheelchair and taken off to the obstetric ward. The father wished her well and took the three-year-old home, not wanting him to be alone. Once home, the father telephoned a few friends in the presence of the three-year-old to tell them about his wife's miscarriage. Eventually, life got back to normal and nothing more was said. Then, seven months later, the same father and his son went to visit some friends. This family's housekeeper had broken a leg and was confined to a wheelchair. The son was absolutely fascinated by this housekeeper in her wheelchair. On the way home after a pleasant visit, the son asked, "How come that house-keeper had a miscarriage?" Initially perplexed, the father suddenly recalled the earlier episode when his son had seen his mother in a wheel-chair. Only then, more than a half a year later, did it become apparent that the child thought a miscarriage was a wheelchair. After all, doesn't a carriage have wheels, and doesn't someone sit in it? To the child it was obvious and logical: his mother had had a miscarriage, and now the housekeeper was sitting in one just like it. I think this example demonstrates how a simple situa-tion can be misunderstood by a child because children see things differently from the way adults do. For this reason, I constantly empha-size that parents should look at a life situation through the eyes of a child, and not expect a child to see the situation through an adult's eyes.

Most parents in preparing their children for the birth of a new sibling assume that they are going to have a single child. Things do not al-ways work out this way either. I have often been approached by parents who have had twins, trip-lets, and even quadruplets. In every instance, the parents assumed that the multiple birth would be particularly confusing to their older child, perhaps even traumatic. I think this assumption is unfair. Most little children have been exposed to some animal, usually a cat, a dog, a hamster, or a pet mouse. These animals all have multiple births, so more than one baby does not seem all that unusual to children. Even if they have not been exposed to animals, children are not as surprised by multiple births as adults.

Unfortunately, parents too often deal with a multiple birth as a "trauma" for an older child. It would be far better if they helped their child regard it as a natural phenomenon. One mother and father who had had triplets consulted me on this very point. The parents expressed concern about how their eighteen-month-old would feel about having three new brothers all at once. To prevent their eighteen-month-old from being "traumatized" they had just about decided to bring the triplets home one at a time, the first baby on one day, the second baby a day later, and the third baby the following day. They planned to handle the situation gradually. When I asked them what they thought their eighteen-month-old would be thinking on the fourth and fifth day, they were confused by my question. I pointed out that he might just begin expecting a new baby each day thereafter for a long time to come. Clearly, this would be far more traumatic than bringing the triplets home together and dealing with the situation honestly in a commonsense way. Can you imagine what might have gone on in the mind of this eighteen-month-old had his parents followed through on their idea? Needless to say, once the parents saw the light, they brought all three babies home together.

-V-

Delivery: The Birth of Your Child

Many women describe giving birth as the greatest, most fantastic experience in their lives, and clearly, every woman who is going to deliver would like to feel the same way. Believe me, that's not always the way it is. I can easily imagine how you must react listening to someone ecstatically describing her marvelous experience while you are feeling nervous or perhaps ambivalent about having your baby, to say nothing of being physically uncomfortable. Even while you are being told about the happiness in store for you, you are bound to feel doubtful and apprehensive. Although the person characterizing her delivery as her most fulfilling experience is really trying to reassure you, wouldn't it be far better to be told the facts about what will happen rather than to hear an idealized version of this imminent and unexperienced event? Learning all you can protects you from feeling that something must be wrong with you if you do not entirely share your friends' enthusiasm. Incidentally, make a note to remember—when you yourself are talking with someone after your child is born—to describe your own experience as one of many and not as the prototype of all childbirth experiences.

The best psychological preparation for delivery includes full knowledge of the delivery procedure, preparation in the form of exercises, training in breathing methods, and, most of all, in not setting up an idealized image of how you want your delivery to take place. If you decide in advance exactly how the delivery is going to occur, any medically necessary deviation from the anticipated pattern can only be viewed by you as a failure on your part. The most disappointed mothers I see are those who tearfully report, "I did all the exercises and was all prepared with the proper breathing. My husband was at my side and coached me, but I couldn't go through with it as I had expected to. I had to take medicine, and I feel as if I failed." Looked at less emotionally, there is absolutely no failure involved, except the mother's failure to fulfill her expectations. In your own case, try not to anticipate exactly how it will be. Just prepare yourself for what is most likely to happen, though you also ought to know a little about unlikely events that could perhaps occur. Many people com-

70

pletely avoid coming to terms with the unexpected in advance because they don't want to make themselves anxious. Actually, knowing all you can might increase your anxiety somewhat, but your knowledge will prevent a feeling of failure from developing if your delivery requires some departure from the usual routine.

It is perfectly understandable that first-time mothers are more likely to be apprehensive about labor and delivery than those mothers who have previously borne children. Obviously, having been through a situation makes the second time around a lot easier. Generally speaking, this is true even if the first delivery was more unpleasant than the mother had originally expected. There are exceptions to this rule, but none of them are mysterious. For example, a mother who had a particularly difficult time with her first child may be far more apprehensive about the birth of her second child than a casual mother approaching the event for the first time. As I have said, a first-time mother's nervousness, uncertainty, and apprehension should lead her to search for as much information as possible about labor and delivery. But I must caution you that in your quest for information you will be highly vulnerable to the opinions and prejudices of others. This is more than understandable. After all, you have no experience of your own.

In your search for information and reassurance as your anxieties periodically surge, don't be surprised when you find people offering information that increases your anxiety rather than information that reduces it. One frantic father called me to discuss his wife's anxiety about her physical activity. Apparently, she had been told that reaching up into a cupboard might cause her to miscarry. Consequently, his wife was afraid to open windows, carry small packages, or even take brisk walks. Her anxiety was compounded by her past history of having had two miscarriages. I told the father to reassure his wife. Her miscarriages were not brought on by reaching for something, and she need neither worry about cupboards nor senselessly restrict her activity.

You will also notice that your feelings are being significantly influenced by past events. You may suddenly recall having heard your Aunt Mildred describe giving birth as an "agony," and you may remember that Aunt Mildred always described her "horror" in hysterical terms. Although you were only ten at the time, as you now recollect her description your anxiety is sure to mount. You may even find it overwhelming, and you may quite properly seek reassurance from some authority. It's only normal to want to find some negation of Aunt Mildred's experience to alleviate your anxiety. Actually, I am convinced your rational reaction to anxiety caused by memories of Aunt Mildred's "horror" is nature's way of making a mother vigilant and concerned about the birth of her child. To alleviate her anxiety, she seeks knowledge, and thus she is better prepared to deal with the normal and natural contingencies of childbirth.

In preparing a couple for childbirth, too many medical professionals forget the fathers. Fathers-to-be have feelings of anxiety and apprehension too, though their worries are usually far less intense than a mother's. To prove this point, I once asked a group of fathers to list their questions about childbirth and give them to me anonymously. Their concerns included what effects giving birth would have on their sexual relations later on, the risks to their wives during childbirth, and how they could learn to feel tenderness toward the expected child. Many a wife gets irritated with her husband during pregnancy because her husband does not seem to be as concerned as she is. She may say, "You don't care at all about having a new baby. You don't even care about me!" Usually such an outburst does not conform to the facts. It simply reflects the discrepancy between the wife's intense feelings, caused in part by her changed physiology, and her husband's less intense reactions and other concerns, which often center on the social, psychological, and economic ramifications. However, it is true that a mother's increased sensitivity can be induced by a marital situation in which she is expected to raise the child practically by herself. Understandably, she may then resent her husband since she will be tied down more than he after the baby is born. But in any case, fathers, as well as mothers, respond to the psychological impact of having a baby. In addition, fathers are usually acutely aware that they will have to share the affections and attentions of their wives with the new baby. Most wives have the same awareness. Many fathers begin to shower their newborn baby with affection, only to encounter a jealous wife, who finds herself feeling that she is unimportant and the baby all-important in her husband's life. Whether it is the mother or father who reacts this way, the reaction is normal and should be dealt with openly and frankly. If the new mother and father have enjoyed the kind of relationship that permits them to avoid the mounting pressure of suppressed emotions by expressing their feelings freely and compassionately, they will be able to deal comfortably with the inevitable frictions caused by the change in the family.

Many parents, after the confirmation of pregnancy and in the weeks prior to delivery, discuss whether or not to try "natural childbirth." To begin with, I say all childbirth is natural! Still, there is a lot of confusion about this term, since it implies that there is something known as "unnatural childbirth." Obviously, given a choice, most people prefer natural childbirth to unnatural childbirth (whatever that means!). Some parents think of trying natural childbirth or the alternative as a choice between pain and no pain. They think that during natural childbirth a mother will get no medication and will suffer considerably. The other method, they think, "knocks out" the mother so that she will miss the entire dreadful experience. I am happy to say that neither expectation is entirely accurate.

What is usually referred to as natural childbirth could better be called prepared childbirth. There are many various techniques for prepared childbirth taught. One of the most popular is the Lamaze method. Other methods vary all the way from teaching fathers how to conduct a delivery at home to simply offering descriptive literature about childbirth. Most commonly, prepared childbirth means that both parents have become familiar with the process of labor and delivery and have learned techniques which facilitate childbirth by minimizing pain, discomfort, and delay. Prepared childbirth also means that the mother has learned how to exercise control of her muscles and breathing in a way that will diminish her discomfort and facilitate her baby's passage through the birth canal. Both parents usually attend classes during the latter part of pregnancy for instruction in prepared childbirth. During actual labor, the father takes an active role in guiding the mother through the breathing and the other exercises she has learned, and at the same time offers her emotional support, assistance, and coaching. In most prepared childbirth methods, the physiology of childbirth is explained and there are opportunities to discuss a parent's emotional concerns. Questions about the details of the delivery itself are encouraged. In most instances, couples visit the labor and delivery rooms. Some classes in prepared childbirth are conducted in a hospital under the direction of the nursing service in conjunction with the department of obstetrics. Others are organized by community-based childbirth-education groups, including the International Childbirth Education Association and the American National Red Cross. Most state and local departments of health have information readily available about these childbirth education programs.

I think it is an excellent idea for parents to elect to try prepared childbirth. Whether or not you eventually have medication to minimize discomfort, knowing the exercises, the breathing patterns, the various phases of labor, and the stages of delivery will be most helpful to you when the time comes. Using the procedures you have previously practiced at the time of delivery will facilitate the birth of your child and may enable you to give birth without medication for discomfort. At the very least, it will certainly minimize the amount of medication necessary. This is beneficial because doctors know that large amounts of sedation given to a mother in labor can cause her baby to become overly sleepy and sluggish.

I must say many parents overemphasize the importance of taking or not taking medication. Some mothers approach delivery with extreme trepidation and anxiety at the thought of any pain. Others approach it with a great deal of bravado, anticipating that they will be able to give birth without experiencing significant pain.

Sometimes they even decide in advance not to accept medication. Since any mother may change her mind when labor actually begins, I think it is more realistic to acknowledge that there will be some pain and that you may want some medication to alleviate the pain. Then again, you may find that you do not. If it turns out that you do, you should not look upon yourself as a failure.

Unfortunately, too many mothers believe that they have failed if they choose to have medication to relieve pain. A mother I spoke to recently, one day after her baby was born, repeated over and over again that she was disappointed with herself because she had requested medication to take the edge off her pain. She was so preoccupied with this point that all the nurses on her floor wondered why she talked about it so much. I finally learned from this woman that she equated no medication with natural childbirth and therefore felt that she hadn't had her child naturally. She found a great sense of relief in my assuring her that her baby had been born naturally, in spite of the medication. This kind of attitude, together with the accompanying feelings of guilt, arises from the misconception that prepared childbirth prohibits the use of any medication at all. It is simply unfair and unnecessary to conceptualize the matter this way.

In my experience, most mothers want to be alert when their baby is born so that they can hear her first sounds and see her immediately after she comes into the world. I would certainly encourage this. If you want to be awake at the moment your baby is born, discuss this seriously with your doctor and see if he or she will try to grant you your wish. I am sorry to say that many doctors think this is unnecessary or foolish and make no effort to consider the mother's feelings. Make sure the person helping you with your delivery intends to respect your wishes in this matter. As a general rule, it is possible for you to be awake at the moment of birth, even if you have medication for pain. Incidentally, while we are discussing doctors, I think it is important for you to discuss the various techniques of prepared childbirth with your doctor after you are familiar with them. Although the doctor's own preference may not be the same as yours, you certainly have the right to make your own choice.

I have discussed elsewhere in this book the importance of getting fathers involved in parenthood right from the start. Specifically, this means getting them involved in understanding all about labor and delivery. They should attend whatever classes the mothers attend, and every effort should be made to have the father present in the labor and delivery rooms. Any birth is a moment of great emotion, and a father who has seen the birth of his own child usually feels exhilarated and excited. Most describe the experience as "Fantastic. I could hardly believe I was seeing my own child come into the world." And a father's presence is important not only for the father himself but for the mother, who needs the father available to her both physically and psychologically.

On many occasions I have watched a new mother and father react to the birth of their child. I cannot tell you how exciting a moment it is for both. The spontaneous remarks I have overheard testify to that. "Oh, my baby! I can't believe it, you're mine, you're mine, I love you, I love you. Please let me hold her. I can't wait," said one mother seconds after her baby was born. Her ecstasy and excitement impressed everyone else in the delivery room. Then after the mother held her baby for a few minutes, the father was given the same opportunity. He exclaimed, "I can't believe that I am holding my own child in my arms. She is mine; I can't believe it; I just want to hold her and take care of her; I can't believe it; I've never been so happy." Remarks like these are common in delivery rooms. I believe they are clear evidence that fathers as well as mothers are prepared to accept responsibility for nurturing their children. The first moments after a baby is born, usually while the family is still in the delivery room, can indeed be a beautiful time to introduce a baby to his or her new family. This introduction becomes the beginning of an important emotional bond, not only between the baby and its parents but also between the mother and father. Observing this particular mother and father after the birth of their daughter, one needed only see their expressions as they looked at each other to understand what happened.

Anyone who has had anything to do with newborns and their parents knows that new parents want to have and evidently need a great deal of contact with their newborns immediately following delivery. Scientific evidence strongly suggests that during the immediate post-partum period, new mothers in particular are highly sensitive to contact or lack of contact with their newborns. One of my own research studies has shown that if there is prolonged post-partum separation between a mother and her child, that mother will handle her baby differently than most mothers who are not subjected to the same kind of separation. And many researchers have studied the same phenomenon in animals. Studies with goats and sheep have demonstrated the importance of bonding at the time of birth: If for as little as fifteen minutes immediately after birth a mother goat has a chance to nuzzle and lick her newborn, she can then pick out her own baby from among a large flock, even if there was a long period of separation after the initial contact. Another study shows that if as little as one hour goes by after a sheep gives birth, and if the mother sheep does not have an opportunity during that time to nuzzle or lick her lamb, the sheep's attachment to the lamb is significantly weakened. As a result, her offspring may be unable to develop normally because of the weakened parent-offspring bond. I know it is risky to generalize from animal behavior to human behavior, but I am convinced that human beings show the same kinds of tendencies toward their offspring following birth.

Unfortunately, many hospitals enforce delivery room procedures which disregard these findings. The normal desire of a new mother to hold her baby and examine it right after birth is not accommodated. The parents whose instincts are ignored then feel guilty about their desires. I believe the parents' natural tendencies should be respected. If for some medical reason they cannot be, mothers suffer greatly. They often experience feelings of depression, anxiety, and failure. These clearly unhappy mothers frequently say, "I don't feel like a mother yet, not until I hold my baby. Only when I hold my baby will I really believe he's mine." I think this reaction indicates that nature has established patterns of behavior in the mother of a newborn baby that make her feel happy in the presence of her baby and anxious if this contact does not take place. I cannot tell you how often I've seen mothers depressed or in tears when they are kept from contact with their new babies because the mother has a slight cold or a slight fever. Any mother is anxious and on edge until she can hold her baby.

Fortunately, more and more hospitals are beginning to modify the procedures surrounding delivery to make it possible for new mothers and fathers to have contact with their new babies as close to the time of birth as possible. Healthy babies are handed to their mothers and then to their fathers moments after they are born. If for some reason it is impossible for a mother to have contact with her baby, perhaps because the baby was born prematurely and had to be immediately placed in an incubator, the hospital procedures encourage contact between parents and their babies as soon as it becomes possible. More and more hospitals are allowing parents of prematures to come into the special-care nurseries where the babies are cared for. Obviously, some antiseptic precautionary procedures have to be observed, but these are easily handled by the nursing staff. Afterward, the parents put their hands in the incubator. They are encouraged to touch their tiny babies and hold them. When they do, many parents are thrilled. I am delighted when a hospital adopts this procedure which openly recognizes the need new parents have for contact with their babies, including premature babies and babies who need some form of special medical care immediately following birth. Parents of these babies should be particularly encouraged to come and visit their babies as often as possible and be close by so that they do not have to suppress their natural, parental instincts.

-VI-

The Hospital Stay

The selection of the hospital where you are going to have your baby will be determined, as a general rule, by the hospital affiliation of your doctor because it is usually not possible to be cared for in a hospital where your doctor does not have a connection. Many prospective parents do not realize the relationship between the doctor, the hospital, the general policies of that hospital, and the kind of care they eventually receive. Consequently, they are sometimes disappointed when they find out, usually when it's too late to do anything about it, that the hospital where their doctor practices will not provide the kind of arrangements they want for their family as a whole. Some hospitals—too many, in my opinion—are very rigid in their procedures. They may not permit fathers in the labor or the delivery room; or they may enforce strict visiting hours; or they may have no facilities which allow a mother to keep her baby in her room; or they may establish an exact feeding schedule that prevents feeding a baby on demand. If you encounter this kind of bureaucratic rigidity (which I myself think of as a kind of institutional hardening of the arteries), you may find yourself becoming agitated, unhappy, angry, or depressed because you are not allowed to act upon your normal and natural tendencies to be close to your baby, to have his father close by in the labor and delivery room, or to become as familiar with your baby as you would like to before taking him home.

All frustrations like these are unnecessary, but not having a chance to get to know your baby is worst of all. You should have enough contact with your baby in the hospital so that you gain confidence and achieve a certain ease in handling your child. Only then are you fortified with enough experience to be able to fend off those relatives and friends who, once you're home, will inevitably suggest that you are not doing things right. If you select a hospital that is flexible and accommodates your wishes about the handling of your child, your positive feelings about parenthood and your confidence will be heightened. If real consideration is given to your desires, you will feel as important as you are entitled to feel. Believe me, nothing will make you feel less important and more angry than being in a hospital that considers its policies more important than its patients' needs. Hospitals with flexible policies will let you have your baby in your room if you want that, will enable your husband to be in the delivery room if you both want him there, and will provide some visiting hours exclusively for fathers so that the mother, father, and baby can be alone together and get to know each other.

What my advice actually boils down to is this: When you select your doctor, find out what hospital affiliation he or she has and find out what the policies of that hospital are before committing yourself to using that doctor. I just cannot tell you how often I have run into new parents who have said, "I wish I had known what that hospital's policies were in advance. We certainly would have gone elsewhere." Others have said, "If I knew my doctor was affiliated with that hospital, I would have chosen a different doctor." As you can see, it is extremely important for you to consider all these matters beforehand so that you may be absolutely sure that, when the time comes, your feelings and your baby's emotional welfare will be dealt with the way you want them to be.

Over the years I have counseled many parents-to-be to do what I have just recommended. Many of them came back to me, reporting that when they inquired about their hospital stay in advance they were accused of being overanxious, picayune, or untrusting. Some doctors do consider it an insult when any patient asks about his or her hospital affiliation. Nevertheless, I think you have every right in the world to ask for this information and to take the response you get into consideration when you make your choice. Any doctor who attempts to make you feel neurotic, or who is insulted by legitimate questions, is simply not the doctor for you. These days it seems midwives perform more and more deliveries. When I ask parents who have selected a midwife rather than an obstetrician why they made that choice, they often report that the midwives seemed to have more compassion and human understanding than the doctors they had met.

Let me counsel you again that it is extremely important for you and your family to be emotionally comfortable and psychologically secure while you're in the hospital. I cannot recommend otherwise. I have seen too many mothers understandably upset by the unwillingness of the nurse on duty to allow them to comfort their crying babies because the nurse thought it was "not time yet." I have seen too many unhappy parents who wanted to be alone with their babies but who were not allowed that privilege because hospital policies prohibited a father's handling his child. I have seen too many mothers having difficulty breast feeding their new babies because they were emotionally upset by not being allowed to see their other children during the hospital stay. As I have said before, in order to establish a good, solid, healthy bond between parents and their babies, it is crucially important to facilitate as much contact as possible in those early hours and days in a way that encourages new parents to feel comfortable with their children. No hospital should put obstacles in the way of expressing your normal, natural desires to be close to your baby and take care of her needs.

Over the years, I have observed a scene that is too common at too many hospitals. A three- or four-year-old child—perhaps even a nine- or ten-year old—stands on the street outside a maternity hospital looking up to an open window, where a waving, smiling mother is trying to reassure the child that she is concerned about him and loves him. The child, tearful and apprehensive, cries, "Mommy, mommy, I miss you. Why can't I come up and see you?" It breaks my heart to see this happen because this kind of separation is inexcusable and unnecessary. This poor child has just become a brother, but he is unable to see the new baby. This is obviously unfair to the child, and it surely does not benefit the mother (which is usually the excuse given for this unfair treatment of the child). Many mothers have told me they have overwhelming and intense desires to have their other children visit them and their new babies. It seems only natural. A few hospitals do allow little children to visit. Invariably, the children are surprised to see their mothers intact and able to get around. They find the surroundings pleasant, and, most important, their mothers' kisses and cuddles tell them that they are still loved. To permit sibling visitation in a maternity hospital simply requires a certain degree of open-mindedness on the part of the professional staff and some consideration for the psychological well-being of the mother, the sibling, and the new baby. In my opinion, human needs should dominate institutions and not the other way around.

One thing you should definitely inquire about is how the hospital will arrange to care for your baby. Some hospitals provide "rooming-in" facilities, which means that a mother may have her baby spend all or most of his time in her room. On the other hand, a lot of hospitals provide no rooming-in arrangements whatsoever. They have a central nursery where the babies stay until they are taken to their mothers to be fed. After they are fed, the babies are returned to the nursery. I must caution you that many a new mother feels thwarted and deprived when the nurse comes and takes her baby away to the nursery. These mothers understand only too well the implication of this procedure, namely that, "The nurse is better equipped to care for the child than his own mother." If you tend to react this way, your confidence can easily be undermined. You may become bored or even emotionally upset. And you would not be the only one. I have observed hundreds of mothers through the windows of a nursery. They always look anxious and their expression always conveys the sentiment, "If I could only hold my baby right now—"

To my mind, the glass barrier between mother and child is inhuman and unnatural.

I must say rooming-in appeals to me because I recommend a great deal of handling, cuddling, and contact with your new baby. It not only gives you a sense of importance but it helps give you the kind of confidence you will need to meet your baby's needs in the future. Rooming-in arrangements vary significantly from hospital to hospital. Some allow a mother to have her baby in her room twenty-four hours a day; others permit having a baby in the mother's room all day but not during the night, when the baby is moved to a central nursery to permit the mother to sleep undisturbed. The nursery nurse takes care of the baby in the middle of the night if he or she wakes up, needing to be held or fed. Almost all rooming-in facilities require that a baby be placed in the nursery during visiting hours. Since the nursery is usually a glass-enclosed room, visitors can see the baby, but they cannot transmit infections because they have no direct contact with the infant. Some rooming-in arrangements require that the baby stay in the nursery for the first twenty-four hours because some hospitals feel that during the first twenty-four hours any baby may require special care. If a baby happens to become congested by some fluid from the delivery that he usually coughs up, he may need to be "suctioned" by a simple, painless device that draws this fluid out of the baby's mouth. Incidentally, the possibility that this special care may be needed is sometimes a good reason for having a baby in a central nursery during the night, even if he spends all day with his mother. During the day, if the mother notices that her baby needs suctioning, she can easily call a nurse. However, as she sleeps at night, she might not be aware that her baby is having difficulty breathing. Consequently, it is not a bad idea to have a baby spend the first few nights in the central nursery where the nurses are right at hand.

In the hospitals that I have visited that offer rooming-in arrangements, the nursing staff usually spends a lot of time answering questions new parents have about handling their babies. Generally, the nurses offer excellent suggestions about how to hold a baby, feed a baby, bathe a baby, and dress a baby. Since the real purpose of the rooming-in program is to bolster parents' confidence, the nurses understand the importance of making themselves available to answer parents' questions and to assist them in any way. One time I remember passing one of the rooming-in units in the hospital when fathers were alone with their wives and babies. To my surprise, I heard an irate father shouting to his wife that she was going to break the baby's neck if she didn't support it properly. Just as I looked in, the nurse explained in a most respectful manner that all babies' heads wobble but that they won't get hurt or come off easily. Nevertheless, the nurse did encourage supporting the baby's head. She handled the matter with dignity and respect for both parents' feelings, particularly the father's deep concern for his daughter's well-being!

Rooming-in arrangements also encourage the kind of early contact between a new father and his family that serves to get fathers really involved in child rearing. The more contact a father has with his baby during the hospital stay, the easier it will be for the whole family when the new baby comes home. If, in the hospital, a father has held his baby, burped his baby, and cared for him in other ways, the father's resulting sense of confidence will give him increased joy in being a parent, and his experience will lighten the load on his wife when she needs help later on. Many hospitals offer classes to mothers on bathing, feeding, and dressing babies during their hospital stay. I think another set of these very same classes should be made available to fathers because I am convinced that it is far better for a hospital to teach these skills to fathers than to expect a new mother to teach the father after the baby gets home. Medical institutions are the ultimate authority in health care. If these prestigious institutions teach mothers but not fathers the arts of feeding, changing, and bathing a baby, their action implies that these activities are female responsibilities. It does not require a great leap of the imagination to see that this practice leads to the idea that all of child rearing is a female, but not a male, responsibility. A hospital that taught fathers these same skills would in effect be saying that child rearing is a father's responsibility too, and, furthermore, the hospital would be conveying the idea that fatherhood is so important that the institution has gone out of its way to set up a program to teach fathers about being fathers. The way it is done now, hospitals tend to ignore fathers, which clearly, and, I think, unwisely, undermines their importance.

During your stay in the hospital, friends and relatives probably will come to visit you. This experience can be as joyous and happy as it can be unpleasant and aggravating. Mostly, you will be proud and excited and thrilled to show off your new baby, but at times you may find that you quickly tire. You may even notice yourself experiencing strange emotions. These reactions are absolutely normal. Many mothers have them, and there is little you can do about them except to respect your feelings and perhaps restrict the number of visitors or limit the duration of their visits. You will also have to prepare yourself for well-meaning friends and relatives who point out odd little things about your baby and in so doing make you anxious or perhaps even panic you. For example, one of them may ask, "Why does the baby's head look so pointed?" in a tone that seems to imply that something is wrong with your baby. Likewise, I recently overheard a visitor standing in front of the glass window of the nursery telling the mother of a two-day-old infant to call the nurse immediately and have her baby's eyes examined. Apparently, this visitor had noticed that the child's eyes were a little crossed as his head turned from side to side. Quite correctly, the nurse pointed out that this is very common in newborns. Then she suggested that if the mother was concerned, she should speak to her pediatrician about it. The visitor turned to the mother as soon as the nurse left and warned, "I'd get that baby out of here right away if I were you. They absolutely don't know anything around here."

Some friends and relatives are secretly envious of you and are, therefore, eager to impress you with their knowledge. If your baby happens to suck one of his hands, one of them might say, "You should stop that this instant so that your baby does not become a thumb-sucker." Now as far as I personally am concerned, thumb-sucking seems to worry too many people much too much. For the first year or more, all babies relate to objects through contact with their mouths. Give any baby a toy, and he immediately puts it in his mouth. This behavior is absolutely normal. Newborn babies, when they accidentally touch their hands to their faces, stimulate the rooting response which causes a baby to open his mouth and begin sucking on whatever is near, usually a finger or thumb. But there is no relationship between this phenomenon and habitual thumb-sucking, despite what your visitor is telling you.

Advice from visitors can be particularly upsetting while you're in the hospital because you are now highly vulnerable to believing anything you hear. You will be inclined to think that other people are right and you are wrong. Visitors often recount their own experiences as gospel, implying that they have more experience than you do and, therefore, that they know best. I often meet a crying mother whose visitors have just left, and I always inquire what the visitors have said. One mother explained to me through her tears how marvelous she had felt and how proud she was that she was going to care for her own baby. She was particularly gratified that her husband had planned to take his allotted vacation to assist her. This couple had decided on their baby's name, and both parents were delighted with their choice. Everything was absolutely fine—until Aunt Isabelle and Uncle Walter arrived. They proceeded to explain how essential it was for the mother and father to have someone else take care of their baby. Aunt Isabelle explained, "You will be tired. You won't be able to handle it. You don't want to get sick, do you? After all, look at what you have just been through. You have to have help!" In spite of this mother's protest that everything was fine, Aunt Isabelle insisted, "All right, you wait! You'll see that I'm right." Uncle Walter then announced that the name they had picked for the new baby was terrible. "The kids in school will tease him with a name like that. You don't want him to grow up to be a sissy, do you? Besides, I know a guy with that name and I can't stand him." This challenge to the parents' choice, with no respect for their feelings, was most unpleasant and psychologically stressing. This poor mother was angry and frustrated. She exclaimed to me, "I know I am right. I know I can care for my baby. I just can't stand being told I am not good enough." As time proved, she was absolutely right. She is an excellent parent and has a marvelously healthy and happy child.

Believe me, there are a lot of Aunt Isabelles and Uncle Walters around, and they are absolutely no help whatsoever. If you encounter them, don't be surprised if you have the kind of reaction this mother had. Because her emotions were so sensitive just after giving birth, she was beginning to fear that she had an emotional problem. I assured her that she was not neurotic and that her emotions were totally understandable. If you have any relatives or friends who are like Aunt Isabelle and Uncle Walter, you may find it better to stave off their visits until you have been home awhile and have been bolstered by some experience. Then you will be able to let their comments and suggestions roll right off your back.

-VII-

Post-Partum Feelings:
Physical or Psychological

In the days, weeks, and perhaps even months after your baby is born, you may notice that you are experiencing some strange and apparently inappropriate emotional reactions. Or you may experience appropriate reactions, but at levels that seem unusually intense. They will vary from feelings of ecstasy and excitement, such as "I never felt so good in all my life" or "I can't believe how tremendously happy having a baby is," all the way to agitation, irritability, or depression—perhaps even occasional thoughts of suicide. Many mothers report having had "the blues" during the week after their babies were born. When this occurs, feelings of heaviness and gloom overwhelm the mother, causing anxiety and despair. Tearfulness is also common.

Strangely, this state seems to occur with no provocation whatsoever. Some mothers who don't get the blues the first week, may get feelings of depression four or five weeks after their baby is born.

Doctors are not really sure what causes post-partum depressions, but they do know that strange feelings occurring around the time of delivery and particularly during the immediate post-partum period are a frequent, and not entirely unexpected, phenomenon. For example, I know one mother who was friendly with and trusted her obstetrician throughout her pregnancy. During her delivery, she was so overwhelmed by her hostility and aggression that she reached out, grabbed her obstetrician's arm as he passed by, and bit him. She was deeply embarrassed by her action, and so, of course, was he. No one came up with an obvious cause for this mother's irrational behavior. Another mother was so ecstatically happy during the five-day period she was in the hospital that she aroused the concern of the nursing staff. They kept saying to me, "We can't understand this woman. She seems almost as if she were high on drugs." When I asked this mother about her fantastic euphoria, wondering if she was indeed taking some drug, she simply said, "I am just high on my baby. I can't get over it, and I'm so thrilled I can't come down." Needless to say, we all relaxed and enjoyed her pleasure.

There really are no typical post-partum depressions. They occur in perfectly well-adjusted, normally happy women who have never been depressed before. For example, one happily married woman had always been able to express her feelings of displeasure toward her husband spontaneously and without feeling guilty. Apparently, her loving relationship with her husband tolerated imperfection. But immediately following the birth of her second child, she suddenly experienced an acute and intense outburst of rage toward him. In a moment of particular anger she screamed, "Get away from me! Don't touch me! I don't want to see you again as long as I live!" Then she began sobbing uncontrollably. Needless to say, this woman startled her husband and upset him. He simply could not understand his wife's reaction since it was totally inappropriate. True, she had been angry at him before, but not for no reason at all. As it happened, his wife's unexplained anger lasted for several days until it finally subsided for reasons as unclear as the reasons it began. Unfortunately, by this time, the husband's reaction to his wife's outburst had become so intense that he was having trouble forgiving her anger. Both agreed to seek help before the situation deteriorated any further. When they consulted a psychiatrist, he proferred the standard psychiatric interpretation: "The wife's reaction was an outburst of repressed hostility toward her husband, primarily caused by her resentment of her pregnancy for which she blamed her husband." This couple's difficulty was regarded as a psychiatric problem in spite of the fact that there was no evidence of any previous marital disturbance or any indication that any emotions had been repressed by husband or wife. In my opinion, a psychiatric diagnosis is questionable in a case such as this one, and others like it, when the event which precipitates the problem is childbirth. I prefer to attribute the intensity of these emotional reactions to the physiological changes that are known to take place during pregnancy and during the post-partum period. I feel the same way about post-partum blues.

During pregnancy there is a slow but marked change in the hormone balance in any mother. During the immediate post-partum period, the hormone changes take place more rapidly. At the very same time, maternal feelings intensify and, among other things, cause a mother to become very protective toward her off-spring. I believe there is a primitive and little understood connection between these hormonal changes and maternal instincts and emotions. I think the physiological changes may very well precipitate the emotional changes. Certainly it is well-recognized that the reverse is true. If a mother begins to experience tension and fatigue while she is nursing, it interferes with the production of milk and the let-down reflex that causes the milk to flow. And it is also known, thanks to a fascinating study, that the hormonal state of a female animal at the time she is presented with her young plays an important part in her reactions. When a lactating female, that is, a female who is producing milk, was presented with a little animal, even if it was not her own offspring, she totally accepted that youngster. If the female was pregnant but not yet lactating, she first attacked the little one, and only then, began to be maternal. If the female was virgin and therefore was neither pregnant nor lactating, she was simply and continuously aggressive and hostile to the little one. This study clearly correlates the maternal reaction of the female to her hormone state at the time. Perhaps, in somewhat the same way, hormones were somehow affecting the woman who bit her doctor.

I know there is no exact parallel between animal and human behavior, but I can accept the idea that part of human behavior is determined by instincts whether or not instinctive reactions are caused by hormonal changes. These instincts, whatever their source, have been refined during the evolutionary process and have become natural tendencies that do help our species survive. Understood in this way, many maternal feelings are actually natural inborn tendencies. If you can accept this concept, you will understand why I encourage you to follow through on your natural tendencies and, whenever possible, to follow the natural way. I trust your instincts, and I think you should too. The lovely, beautiful, and spontaneous feelings that mothers have while feeding babies; the anxiety mothers feel when they hear a baby cry; the special closeness a mother feels when her baby stares at her face—all are examples of natural tendencies that help children, and the species, survive.

On the other hand, it is not uncommon for a mother to get a strong sense of wanting to reject her child within a few days after her baby is born. She may first notice this feeling during one of those quiet moments when she has a chance to look over her baby all by herself. She finds herself thinking, "He is so ugly. How did I get myself into this? He didn't turn out the way I thought he would. I don't even want to touch him. I think I would like to get dressed, leave the hospital quietly, not tell anyone where I am going, and never be heard from again." Most mothers, when they have these momentary desires to reject their babies, feel horribly guilty. Generally, they quickly reach out, pick up their babies, hold them close, and say, "Oh, how could I feel that way about you, such a lovely little boy, my own baby!" The mother's guilt, caused by that moment of rejection, most often causes a mother to give her baby a little extra cuddling, if only to prove to herself that she doesn't really dislike her child. I am sure her feelings of rejection were real, and I am also sure that her feelings of remorse are real. My point is that the whole sequence leads to an additional little hug, a little bit more cuddling than the baby might otherwise have gotten. Perhaps this is another of nature's ways of making absolutely sure a baby gets the kind of love and affection he absolutely needs.

Incidentally, most mothers are understandably reluctant to confess that they momentarily do not want their babies. They fear that someone will consider them unfit for parenthood, or worse, brand them as needing psychiatric help. But in my classes with new mothers, I find that at least half of them acknowledge—if only with smiles—that they have experienced these feelings, usually within the first few days after the birth of their child. My mentioning and implying that it is common enough to comment on seems to reassure them. Believe me, ambivalent feelings toward newborns, or toward any child, for that matter, are very common. During the post-partum period, this is particularly true since the fluctuation from positive to negative can be quite extreme. Fortunately, the strong feelings of love and protection generally seem to dominate.

Mothers who are subjected to severe marital tension or emotional stress during pregnancy sometimes begin not to want to have a baby. Often, these intense emotions are thought to be the cause of a miscarriage or a series of miscarriages. Studies dealing with rats and mice have shown that when a pregnant female is placed under stress, her body tends to "absorb" the growing embryo into itself and thus prevent the baby from being born. Clearly, the stress reaction is what causes this to happen. In some instances, doctors have attributed premature delivery to emotional stress. Existing clinical evidence supports this idea, and I am inclined to agree. I think it might be nature's way of preventing a child from being born into a family situation that is not good for his healthy emotional development.

The more negative a mother feels about having a child in the first place, the more this factor will interact with her body's physiological changes which in turn influence the severity of her ambivalent reactions. I often see a mother who is experiencing many family problems or emotional tensions undergo a post-partum reaction marked by serious depression, agitation, and irritability. Having a child is clearly a burden to her, and the additional demands caused by the birth of her child serve only to stress an already stressful situation. After all, now that she has had the baby, she is, in a sense, stuck. She will not be able to move around as freely as she might like, her financial burdens will be higher, her baby will be very time consuming, and she has the responsibility for another human being's life.

For example, I was once asked to speak with a mother who had just given birth to her first child. The doctors and nurses reported to me that she either took an irrationally protective attitude toward her daughter or she seemed absolutely detached from her and totally "tuned out." This mother's overprotective reaction was so extreme that she seemed to be rescuing her daughter from some actual harm, yet there was no real danger at hand. After speaking with her and learning some of the tragic events that had taken place in this mother's life, I could see that her overprotectiveness was directed against her own intense but sporadic feelings of rejecting her child. This mother's husband, whom she loved dearly, became acutely ill and died when she was six months pregnant. She herself had no living relatives except a brother who was handicapped and dependent on her. She had few savings and now had to rely upon herself as the sole support of her brother, herself, and now her child. Actually, she wanted her baby, but real events in her life forced her to feel overwhelmed by her new and added responsibility. Marked ambivalence or even a negative reaction on the part of such a mother is quite understandable.

Although I am inclined to believe that many persistent and unrelenting post-partum depressions may be due to a basically negative attitude to having a child in the first place, I am absolutely sure that wanting the baby does not preclude periodic feelings of anger, hostility, and rejection, even in emotionally healthy parents. An example of what I mean is what some of us call the "drop the baby out of the window syndrome." Some mothers experience this feeling when the baby is a month or two old, sometimes even later in the child's life. A parent totally frustrated by his child wonders if the solution to his problem is to drop his child out the window. Although the extent of the reaction is usually not so extreme, feelings of frustration caused by the responsibilities of child care often periodically overwhelm parents. They do so because parental responsibilities and the problems parents cope with are very real. Recognizing this is the first step toward coming to terms with your feelings of frustration when they occur. If you deny these feelings, or attribute them to emotional problems, you will only feel guilty. You may then repress your feelings and at some other time they could erupt so forcefully that you could not control them. It's far better to know that having a child is at times a burden and that you may have momentary impulses to hurt your baby. Even good parents are exposed to these periodic feelings since they occur in all parents. But if you should find yourself unable to control these impulses, you should seek professional help immediately. There is nothing unusual about occasionally wanting to wring your child's neck, but you mustn't do it.

The expected outcome of any pregnancy is a wanted, healthy, live child with whom the mother can have immediate contact. Consequently, an interruption in a pregnancy due to a miscarriage or a clinical abortion, which purposely terminates the pregnancy, usually leads to a period of depression. This sadness, which is normal, can even be expected. I have observed many patients who have had miscarriages or abortions and then experienced transitory depressions, sometimes even grief. But I have never noticed any long-range emotional problems resulting either from clinical abortions or spontaneous miscarriages. Consequently, I tend to attribute the woman's depression and her feelings of emptiness to physiological changes that necessarily occur when her pregnancy is terminated. On the other hand, I have also observed women who delivered a baby they could not or did not want to raise, usually because they were unwed and had become pregnant by accident. Some decided to give their babies up for adoption; some did not. Many of the mothers whose children were adopted by someone else were plagued for years by nightmares about their children; others were later desperate to find their children and take them back. Some mothers who decided to keep their unwanted children later experienced a severe emotional disturbance or mental breakdown. From a strictly psychological point of view, I think early termination of an unplanned pregnancy by clinical abortion is far less devastating psychologically to all involved than allowing the pregnancy to go to term, and giving birth to an unwanted child. Rearing a child in an institution because his parents refuse him, or raising a child whose parents consciously or unconsciously reject him, all too often leads to the kind of human suffering that is immeasurable. Naturally there are exceptions to this general rule. Consequently, I always recommend that all the possible ways of dealing with the problem should be completely explored by the pregnant woman, her family, and her doctor. Incidentally, the mother herself should be given every chance to decide what should be done in the best interest of everyone involved. Of course, the most satisfactory approach to this problem is to prevent it arising in the first place. Since a large percentage of unwanted pregnancies occur because of ignorance about reproduction and birth control, educating people can help minimize the human suffering that usually accompanies unwanted pregnancies. But not until society elevates the status of parenthood can we be absolutely certain that all our children are wanted.

-VIII-

Handling Advice from Others

As your visitors in the hospital have already begun to teach you, there is something about a parent with a newborn baby that motivates all kinds of people, including total strangers, to offer you plenty of unsolicited advice. They will caution you about all sorts of potential dangers and tell you how to protect yourself and your child from all kinds of impending disasters. I can't tell you how many times I have been approached by strangers when I was walking on the street with my own children during their early years. Without hesitation these good citizens cautioned me about the hazards of the toys my children had with them or explained the consequences of dressing children as irresponsibly as they felt I had or warned me that my running son might fall and seriously injure himself. Who are these people who give you so much advice and so little real help? And what is their motivation? Sometimes you wonder why they don't mind their own business. Eventually, you may even begin to get the feeling that people like this are out to get you, and you are probably correct. I think they are really envious of you and unconsciously want to undermine the pleasure you are having with your child. I have often joked that they are basically repressed kidnappers. Although I don't really mean that, it does seem as if they are trying hard to take away the satisfactions of parenthood and the pleasures of childhood all at the same time.

If I am amazed at the freedom with which advice is given, I must say I am more amazed at the advice itself. And it does not seem to make much difference whether the advice comes from friends, relatives, strangers, concerned others, or from various health professionals, most specifically physicians, pediatricians, psychologists, and psychiatrists. In many instances, the advice is simply and plainly wrong. And often the advice-givers' attitude is what I must call "anti-parent" in that it undermines any pleasure, satisfaction, or confidence that a parent may have. Let me illustrate: When a mother feeds her newborn for the first time and notices her infant looking straight into her face while suckling the breast or the bottle, that new mother experiences a warm and exciting feeling. Invariably, she smiles because she is deeply gratified by the baby's eye contact with her face. When I ask new mothers to confirm this, they grin happily when they recall that situation. They remember wondering, "Does my baby know me? I feel like it's the beginning of our relationship." This is a normal and natural reaction as a new infant fixates on her mother's face. The exhilarated mother, usually wanting to share her happiness at this moment, calls someone over and says, "See, my baby is looking at me!" The nurse or doctor, often in an officious or detached manner, simply says, "Not possible. Your baby can't see yet." Then the dismayed parent is told that a baby can't see until two weeks, or three weeks, or four weeks, or six weeks, or eight weeks of age (the length of time cited depends solely upon where the professional was trained). Now the fact is that a newborn baby does see and does tend to look directly into the face of the person who is feeding her. So not only is the information the medical professional proffered erroneous but it specifically contradicts what the mother has just experienced. Worse, it tends to debase the capabilities of a newborn baby and minimize the importance of the warm and dramatic experience the mother just had. This kind of unfounded advice detracts from the pleasures you will get from your infant. That's why I call it "anti-parent." Why would a newborn look a mother straight in the face immediately upon suckling to the breast or bottle if the mother's face was not an object of importance? Why doesn't the baby look elsewhere? This experience in and of itself tells me that a baby is not only capable of seeing, but is capable of associating his mother's face with the pleasure that is about to take place in the feeding process. Laboratory studies have quite clearly shown that babies under two days of age spend more time looking at complicated visual patterns than plain surfaces, even if the plain surfaces are brightly colored. These same studies demonstrate that babies prefer faces and concentric circles like bull's-eye targets to other kinds of patterns, such as horizontal lines or checkered squares. It seems as if the newborn actually seeks out more complicated visual patterns.

A new mother telling a nurse that her baby just looked her straight in the face during his first feeding will sometimes be informed that a newborn can see only shapes and shadows. Any new mother's immediate interpretation of this statement is, "My baby is not looking at me." But if you really analyze the nurse's comment, you will soon realize that any face is only a shape and a series of shadows! What else is visual experience but seeing shapes and shadows? Again, the nurse is undermining the warm feeling the mother experienced and demeaning the importance of the early mother-child relationship. Another gratifying moment for any new parent is when his baby first smiles. Generally, the excited parent turns to some professional and says, "Look! My baby is smiling!" More often than not, the professional answers, "No, No! That's not a smile. That's gas!" Well, I am absolutely appalled at that conclusion. I know gas does not make me smile, and I am sure it doesn't make you smile. Neither does it make a baby smile. Why should gas cause a smile any more than a smile causes gas! I think the notion that gas makes a baby smile developed a long time ago when some baby smiled and coincidentally passed gas at the very same moment. Some professional who was observing immediately concluded that the gas caused a smile. The observation was then transmitted as gospel from person to person until it was so generally accepted that no one questioned it. Many ridiculous and unfounded bits of information have been accumulated and passed on in this way.

/ Let's examine other kinds of advice that new parents get. You will find that when your baby cries, you will have a strong desire to pick up the baby, find out what is causing him to cry, and make him happy. This is a perfectly normal and natural desire, probably an inborn behavior pattern that helped the species survive. Wait and see what happens when you exercise this natural tendency! You are sure to find someone saying, "Uh-uh, uh-uh, don't pick up that baby. You'll spoil it!" Needless to say, your desire to do what is best for your newborn will leave you vulnerable to their advice, particularly if your advisor is a doctor or nurse or experienced friend. After all, you don't want to spoil your newborn baby. Unfortunately, once the erroneous advice is given, you are bound to be anxious no matter what you do. If you follow the advice, you will be unhappy suppressing your natural instincts. Conversely, if you follow them, despite what you've been told, you may feel guilty and worry that you are in fact spoiling your child. Since you were more comfortable before the advice was proffered, perhaps you should ignore it. In this case, I know you should. The advice not to pick up your crying baby, in effect, says, "Your baby will be better off being unhappy than if you pick him up and make him happy." If you look at it this way, the recommendation will seem as foolish as it is.

Many people state that picking up a crying baby will make the child want to be picked up every minute of the day. In my way of thinking this proposition is ridiculous. If I were to advise you against having lunch when you are hungry for fear that the satisfaction that comes with eating would lead you to eat, and eat, and eat, and eat until you burst, you would think I was crazy. The fact of the matter is that eating makes your hunger go away so that you can concentrate on doing something else. Similarly, satisfying a baby's infantile need to be held and comforted makes that need go away so that the baby can proceed with other tasks in his or her early development. Fortunately, the average parent disregards advice that picking up a baby when she cries will spoil her. Unfortunately, though, the mother or father who disregards the advice is often ridiculed as a "neurotic parent." When this happens you are really being told that you are emotionally disturbed because you try to make your baby happy. What can possibly be more "anti-parent" than that!

The next line of offense from relatives, friends, and concerned others about picking up a crying baby is generally, "You shouldn't do that. Crying is good for the lungs!" Now there is absolutely no scientific evidence to support this conclusion. Many babies who cry very little as babies turn into children whose lungs function just fine. Therefore, I always counter this advice by saying that if crying is good for the lungs, then bleeding must be good for the veins. Both statements are equally ridiculous! Hopefully, when this particular suggestion is made, you will be strong enough to follow your natural tendencies to make your baby happy and disregard the "anti-parent" advice.

I am absolutely against letting a baby "cry it out." However, if your baby, during his early months, tends to cry at bedtime, or if he experiences bouts of crying at other times, eventually someone—your pediatrician, another professional, or possibly a friend—will recommend that you "Let your baby cry it out." Believe me, this is common advice and is even endorsed by some esteemed child-care experts. They feel that letting a baby cry it out will teach the baby not to expect you to be there every time he wants you. Letting a helpless infant cry it out may very well teach him that. He may indeed learn that you will not be there when he needs you. But what you have taught him can be seriously detrimental to his healthy emotional development.

The resources of an infant to cope with stress are rather primitive and limited. If you deliberately let your child cry for an extended period, your child may be unable to cope with the excessive stress you have created without "going off to sleep" or "tuning out the world." Using these primitive defense mechanisms is his only way of relieving stress and discomfort unassisted. If these particular defense mechanisms are used constantly, a child adopts this pattern as his primary means of coping with any stress. Most of us know adults who use this type of defense by withdrawing into sleep, by never noticing what's going on, or by denying reality by overdrinking or by using some other means that "tunes out" the world. These individuals react as if they are helpless and unable to use their own resources to eliminate their discomfort. Perhaps they were taught this as crying babies.

I am often asked how parents can be sure that their pediatrician is giving them good advice about their child's behavior and their emotional reactions to the child's behavior. The answer is it's very hard to be sure. Too many people assume that a pediatrician who has passed his or her board-certification examinations knows all about human behavioral development. This assumption is just not accurate at the present time, though there seems to be some interest in increasing pediatric training in child-rearing practices. For the present I can only recommend that you be wary of pediatricians who tend to undermine your confidence, downgrade your natural tendencies, give advice without explaining the basis for their advice, or imply that you are neurotic. Your pediatrician, like your obstetrician, should be "askable" if you have questions about your child's behavior.

I am always amazed at the number of people in the child-development and parent-education fields who consciously or unconsciously transmit the idea that newborn babies are not able to learn or respond in a meaningful way. Week after week I have to counter this impression in my discussions with new parents. Just recently six new mothers out of a group of eleven insisted that they had been told by respected professionals that their babies didn't know what was going on around them. Nothing is further from the truth. Newborn babies are highly responsive to their environment, and they are quite capable of learning. Studies have clearly shown that babies begin to make associations between their experiences and their feelings in the first days of life. In my own behavioral research laboratory, we have been able to demonstrate that as early as the third day of life babies are able to recognize a given musical tone, and that within a matter of minutes the babies' familiarity with that tone can be documented. While it is very hard to measure the exact degree to which a baby is responding, simply because she has few ways to communicate her responses, it is not at all hard to prove that she receives information and records it in her brain. We also have proved that newborn babies need stimulation. They like to have things to look at and they like to hear, feel, smell, taste, and experience a sense of movement. This desire for stimulation is a primitive forerunner of later, more complicated learning, but is nevertheless learning.

I frequently hear it said that parents are not all that important in raising children, and that others can do the job just as well. I totally disagree. It is just not possible to duplicate the fascinating configuration of inborn tendencies in a newborn infant and the natural parental inclinations that mesh with them to provide gratification for the infant and his parents at the same time. The baby acts, the parent reacts, and the baby reacts to the reaction of the parent in a symbiotic cycle. For example, when a hungry newborn cries, his parent naturally tends to pick him up. The baby's discomfort, which causes him to cry, also gives him an increased desire to suck. Simply touch a baby's cheek gently, close to the mouth, when he is hungry, and you will find that he turns in the direction of the touch, opens his mouth and begins to suck vigorously on whatever object happens to be close at that time. At about the same time that her baby begins to cry, his mother is probably beginning to notice some discomfort in her breasts as the large supply of milk causes them to become engorged. If she follows her natural tendency to pick the baby up, she most probably holds him near her breasts. If her breast touches the baby's cheek, the baby will move in the direction of the touch, search for something to satisfy his suck-

ing need, which because of the physical prox-
imity will most likely be his mother's nipple.
While the baby sucks at his mother's breast to
satisfy his own sucking needs, he will simultaneously relieve his mother's discomfort. While her
baby is feeding, the mother will express her
pleasure with her baby by touching him, smiling
at him and talking to him in a way that provides
the proper stimulation needed for the baby's
healthy emotional growth. In response, the baby,
who looks the mother straight in the face, will
begin to associate the gratification of his sucking
needs and the diminution of his discomfort with
his mother's face, smell, taste, and voice. When
the baby is through feeding, he will relax totally
as he goes off to sleep. When this occurs, many
babies retract their facial muscles and smile.
When the baby smiles, his parent invariably
smiles back, almost in a reflex manner. This
whole rather lovely interaction clearly leads to
the development of a bond between mother and
baby that helps the baby become dependent in a
healthy way upon the very people who are most
likely to care for him since they are the same
ones who were responsible for bringing him into
this world.

It is a constant surprise to me that the
beautiful quality of the natural instincts that
cause parents to respond to their babies' needs is
constantly undermined. Parents who pick up
crying babies are not neurotic, nor are they
spoiling their children, or interfering with the
development of healthy lungs. And mothers who

enjoy eye-to-eye contact with newborns and take pleasure in the smile that occurs when the baby's sucking need has been gratified do not need to be told they are the effects of gas. The point is that natural tendencies on the part of parents do not have to be instilled. They just have to be respected by you and by anyone who gives you advice.

A lot of unsound advice is transmitted not only by friends and professionals, but by the parents of new parents as well. Ironically, these are the very people who should have the most interest in supporting you and your offspring. But many new grandparents find it difficult to think of their child, who is now a parent himself, as anything but a youngster who is not yet mature enough to undertake the responsibilities of parenthood. The grandparents think their child is not sufficiently knowledgeable to be a parent unless he is given all kinds of advice. Unless a certain degree of independence from parents has already been achieved, it is extremely hard for any new parent to resist this kind of pressure from grandparents. Nevertheless, if you have not gotten your parents to recognize and accept your individuality, this is the time to insist they do. If you do not, it will be extremely hard for you to raise your own child with a sense of self-confidence and for your own child to have a sense of trust in you and respect you as an individual.

One father I know used to call his mother each evening at 6:30. After the usual amenities, she would inquire about his baby. Almost daily she gave advice, aroused anxiety, and insisted that her son call the pediatrician to validate her concerns. Although he always maintained that she didn't influence him a bit, his subsequent remarks generally indicated quite the opposite. He usually did call the pediatrician, who most often reassured him that all was well. This father would then call his mother and report what he had been told. This father was still unconsciously turning to his mother for help, and she was complying with his request for assistance. So, in a way, she was raising the child and not the father.

If your parents do not accept your independence and continually insist on advising you, you should be prepared to follow through on your own natural tendencies. Grandparents need not act exactly like parents nor deal with their grandchildren precisely the same way the parents do, but they must not undermine the integrity of the parents. I do not mean that grandparents' advice should always be ignored, but I do think it is important that new parents acknowledge their own natural tendencies and follow them. Even if they sometimes make mistakes, it's still better than having to rely upon the grandparents to make the decisions about the rearing of the children.

Recently, the mother and father of a three-year-old came to me, deeply concerned about the way their child was reacting to being left alone with his maternal grandmother. The child was often anxious and clung to his parents, frequently woke up with nightmares, and said he wanted to stop using the toilet and go back to wearing diapers. These parents told me that the maternal grandmother, who lived in the same building as they did, was a deeply anxious person. They said she was constantly pointing out all the possible disasters that might befall their child if they did not heed her warnings. The grandmother was clearly one of those people who sees danger everywhere. She would grab up the child when he was wandering along on the street and happened to come close to a stranger because she feared his being kidnapped. She would not let the child play with other children because she feared that another child might hurt him. She constantly washed his hands because she feared unnamed germs. The child's parents recognized the grandmother's irrational behavior, generally ignored her advice, and handled things pretty much the way they wanted to. But their child was defenseless when his grandmother panicked. The youngster began to be anxious because he felt his grandmother wanted him to be anxious. He was victimized by her perception of the world. Consequently, he clung to his parents and began acting like a helpless baby so that he would be cared for and protected by them. It was clear to me that this youngster had to be protected from his "well-meaning" grandmother and at the same time had to spend more time with his own parents. Perhaps it's an unusual example, but I have selected it because it shows that parents, and not grandparents, are the proper people to raise children.

-IX-

The Practicalities of Life with a Newborn

Bringing your baby home for the first time is indeed an exciting event which evokes special feelings for the mother, father, and everyone else involved. It will be particularly exciting if you are a new parent, because for the first time you will be completely on your own. You will no longer have the hospital staff, doctors, or nurses around to make decisions for you, and you will not have to conform to established routines. In a way, being alone in your own home is a relief, but in another way, it is scary. In spite of all the preparations you made before going to the hospital, you will undoubtedly find that some things do not work out exactly the way you planned. Your disappointment about this may make you feel disorganized and inadequate, but the fact that things do not turn out the way you thought they would is perfectly normal. In this way, coming home is a little preview of how life with a baby will continue to be.

Day-to-day life with a newborn baby will be quite a departure from what your life was like before. While everyone knows this intellectually, the reality still comes as a shock when you are actually faced with the practicalities. To begin with, your time will be less your own now than it ever was. And you will have more to do than ever before. Whether you are planning a brief one-hour visit with a friend, or a prolonged visit involving several nights away from home, you will find yourself preoccupied with your baby's welfare. It will be difficult to go anywhere without first organizing all sorts of paraphernalia you think you may need. "Do I have diapers?" "Have I brought an extra blanket?" "Have I packed a little toy?" "Do I have the baby's bottle?" (This is never a problem for a mother who breast feeds.) When everything the baby could use is organized, you may find that you have completely forgotten your house keys. That's only human. After all, you can't remember everything all the time!

Having a baby in your home requires a maximum of flexibility, a lot of energy, and great patience. Although some of your plans and preparations may go down the drain, I still think it's a good idea to make those plans. It really is helpful to have some general idea about how you plan to cope with your baby's care. I remember one mother who was expecting her second child consulting with me about bringing her new baby home. She had spent a lot of time getting organized. She planned to devote her attention to her older child when the baby was asleep, and she had prepared activities to keep her older child busy while she breast fed the baby. Everything, she thought, was perfectly planned, and, in her opinion, she was headed for a resounding success. Although I commended her efforts to get organized in advance, I also suggested that she not be disappointed if things did not work out exactly the way she expected them to. I did not want to undermine her confidence, but I did want her to realize that things might not work out according to plan. If they happened not to, I was anxious that she should not consider herself a failure. So I emphasized flexibility as much as I could. Being the well-organized person she was, she had to plan things systematically. I felt I could not actively discourage her from being organized, for that would be asking her not to be herself. Advising a person to act in a way that is contrary to her nature and personality often leads her to feel inadequate. So I praised her planning, counseled flexibility, and repeatedly reassured her that she had what it took to deal with the situation. What I was trying to do was to get her to accept the possibility that her plan might have to be altered and, further, to recognize that she would not be a failure as a parent if her plan happened to change. Three weeks after her baby was born, this mother telephoned me, delighted and happy with her newborn. She was exuberant about the way she was handling the situation. She then admitted that she had felt insecure before her baby was born. In retrospect, she recognized that all her organizing was really her way of dealing with her own anxiety. She admitted that things did not work out the way she had planned, and she was thankful that I had emphasized the need for flexibility.

Thousands of new parents have taught me that many people never realize beforehand what having a new baby at home will be like. Some admit, "Had I known what it would be like, I really think I would not have had children at all. I really love my sleep and my privacy, and I didn't realize how much a baby could change them." Others say, "It never occurred to us that we would not be able to go to a movie without making intricate plans for a baby-sitter." Or, "Having people over is no longer as simple as it used to be." Apparently, parents like these never asked what parenthood would be like. Certainly, no parent ever told them.

Being physically and emotionally exhausted is by no means an uncommon experience for a new parent. Since the whole process can be very tiring, it is a wise idea for a mother not to try to do the job all alone. You might get overly exhausted, depressed, and angry. You see, the more fatigued you become, the more irritated it makes you, and this irritation feeds back to your baby, causing him to be more irritable, which simply increases your own discomfort, and so on. A downward cycle is set in motion and it can only be broken by arranging to share the responsibility of meeting your baby's needs. That's why I think it's essential that both parents share the work of caring for their baby. They can relieve each other as the fatigue level mounts.

I must warn you that there will be times when you wonder if your baby is worth all the trouble. You will be tempted to ignore her so that she will learn that you won't always be around to wait on her. Don't give in to that temptation. You only run the risk that your baby will develop a pattern of fussing as a way to greet you. Studies show that unresponsive parents eventually have to cope with infants who fret merely at the appearance of a parent. This result is obviously quite the opposite of what you intend to accomplish if you follow the advice of others who tell you that you are spoiling your baby. Of course, you will have many moments of ambivalence— wishing that you had never gotten yourself into this situation in the first place and then wanting desperately to do everything you can to make that young life contented, comfortable, and happy. Your quite normal desire to be with your baby and care for him will be criticized, sometimes vociferously, by others. But if new parents did not have an overwhelming desire to protect their children, how could the species ever have survived?

The questions most frequently put to me by parents who are about to take their new baby home or who have just taken a baby home are these: "What should we do about the baby waking up at night? Should the baby sleep in our room or in its own room? Should we put the baby in a large crib or a small bassinet? Should the baby share a room with his brother or sister, or is it better for us to keep the baby in our room? Is there anything wrong with giving the new baby our older child's crib and moving him into a big bed so that he will feel bigger and more important?"

If there ever was a true statement, this is it: "Babies wake up at night!" Most babies wake up a number of times each night during the first few months. New parents understandably feel that all the world is sleeping and that they are the only ones awake. "No one told us our baby would wake up four, five, or even ten times at night. My neighbors keep telling me that we must be having a problem. Is that true?" The answer is no. It is very common for a newborn to wake up many times during the night and each time interfere with the sleep of both parents. This can be very aggravating and may try your patience enormously, since one parent or the other has to get up, see what's making the baby cry, and get him back to sleep. Ideally, both parents should share this responsibility, but often this job becomes the mother's. The rationale is that she does not have a regular job, unlike the father who must get up the next morning and spend the day working. This approach too often results in a fatigued and irritable mother who resents being the one who has to wake up and take care of the baby. One couple I know decided to share the responsibility. They worked the problem out successfully by arranging two six-hour shifts; one parent took the 9 P.M. to 3 A.M. shift, and the other took the 3 A.M. to 9 A.M. shift. They alternated shifts to equalize the amount of sleep each had in the course of a night. No matter how you and your spouse organize it, you are bound to feel that your baby's waking up in the night will never ever end. And all the while, your friends, relatives, and neighbors can be counted on to imply that their babies sleep through the night and that all their children always did. More than likely, they are not telling the truth. The fact is that, sooner or later, your baby will sleep through the night. Until then, when he cries, you must find out what is bothering him, fix it, and help him get back to sleep.

As a general rule, if you have an extra room for a new baby, you ought to have the baby use that room right from the start. This arrangement tends to protect your privacy. It is better for you in the long run, even though the parent whose turn it is to get up at night to care for the baby has to walk a longer distance. There is another reason I recommend that your baby have his own room. Letting a baby live in your room while an older child is living in his own room is often resented by the older child, who can only feel that the little baby is getting preferential treatment. Because the new baby is so dependent on his parents, he is, in fact, getting one kind of preferential treatment, so the older child has a point. Whether your older child and the new baby share a room depends, of course, on the number of rooms you have available. If you do have a room available for each child, use them. Older children like their privacy as much as you do, and they worry that a baby will invade their domain and take it over completely. This concern causes an older child to protect his own bed, his own toys, and all of his other possessions. For the same reason, you should avoid taking things from your older child and giving them to the baby. If they are babies' toys your older child really doesn't want, remember to ask his permission before you give them away to your baby.

A newborn does not necessarily need a crib. You might try putting her down to sleep in a carriage. A carriage can be readily moved from room to room, which can be very convenient, and it can be rocked gently back and forth to help your baby go to sleep. Actually, a baby will care more about being wrapped snugly or swaddled tightly than the size of her bed. If you are planning to have your new baby use your older child's crib, get a regular bed for your older child and let her make the transition to sleeping in it a few months before the new baby is born. Remember to remove the crib from the older child's room. When the time comes to put the baby in the crib, consider repainting it, or redecorating it in some other way that makes it look different than when it was used by your older child.

After the baby comes home, you can expect

a number of visitors. You will be happy to see many of them, but some visitors tend to be overwhelming, and you may not want to see them. You may even have times when you feel that you want no one around. Don't hesitate to ask your friends and relatives to respect your feelings. At first, you may find that you are nervous about letting a lot of different people handle your child. It will not hurt your child, but don't be bashful about explaining to your visitors that you would prefer to let them hold your baby during a later visit, after you and he have gotten more used to each other.

When a new baby comes home, the families of each parent sometimes become competitive and vie with each other for time with your baby. This in-fighting can be very taxing. If it gets out of hand, both mother and father may have to be very firm about enforcing visiting hours if you are not to lose control over your life. Over and over again, in my classes for new parents, this problem arises: How does one regulate visits from relatives without offending them? One father described his unsuccessful attempts to keep his brother's wife from inviting herself over. He had tried not answering the phone, but this approach made things even worse. Since no one answered the telephone, she assumed something was wrong and rushed over immediately. I suggested to him, as I have to numerous other parents, that he and his wife should not place themselves in the position of trying to avoid people or constantly having to make excuses. Instead, I suggested they take the initiative, call the sister-in-law and ask her if she would like to come to visit. Naturally, she will be delighted by the invitation and will say, "Yes, of course." Then, you can then say, "Wonderful, I will call you back and let you know when it is a good time. Today isn't good but I'll get back to you soon." In this way you are offering the chance to visit and yet you yourself are controlling when it will take place. Your anxious visitors will have their invitations, but they simply have to wait for you to tell them when to come. Generally, this works much better than trying to avoid the situation by making excuses. After all, how many excuses can you make?

Although you may risk offending your relatives whatever procedure you adopt, you will at least be protecting the integrity of your marital relationship and your feelings about each other. Believe me, your relationship will need some protecting. The first month with a new baby is like a "shake-down." All the weaknesses in a marriage begin to emerge and the sensitivities of each parent are very noticeable. I remember one new mother who came to see me shortly after the birth of her first child. She had already learned that she and her husband no longer had the privacy they were used to when they lived alone. She had found out that they seldom sat down to dinner and got through it without interruption. The few times they had managed to do so were cherished events. She mentioned that she had had to change her schedule and even the nature of the food she served. Prior to her baby's birth, the meals she prepared for her husband were elaborate. Having a baby at home made it difficult if not impossible to prepare meals the way she wanted to, and often she and her husband had to eat leftovers. She pointed out how tired she was toward the end of the day and how much she wanted to rest, but she always had to rush to get the house cleaned and dinner cooked. She was aware of her husband's increasing jealousy and envy of the baby and was working hard to minimize it. But as supportive and warm as her husband was, and as excited as he was about being a father, he apparently couldn't help remarking now and then, "We haven't had a decent meal since that [pause] baby was born." When this mother consulted me she was upset. She felt that her husband did not realize how little time she had either to herself or to prepare for his daily homecoming. He had even gone so far as to say that she was disorganized. I told this mother that irritability and marital conflict are common after a baby comes home from the hospital. I also told her that the need for continued closeness between husband and wife would never be greater and that, unfortunately, the realities of everyday life with the newborn baby would tend to interfere with this need. I suggested that if she persevered, things would get better as the baby got older, particularly if she and her husband made an effort to discuss their jealousies and feelings of resentment in a constructive way that just might lead to a solution of their problems.

Needless to say, the best way to prepare a marriage for the stress of having a baby is to have a good marital relationship in the first place. Both husband and wife will find it easier if they have achieved their individuality and independence, and if they do not need continued reassurance from one another to maintain a healthy confidence. Of course, it is crucially important that the communication between husband and wife be open so that they can discuss their feelings before resentment builds up. It also helps to recognize in advance that a lot of rearranging of time, space, and priority will have to take place in your life to make room for a baby and, at the same time, maintain your marital equilibrium. It's not easy, but it can be done.

People often overlook one significant factor in considering the stress that having a baby puts on a marriage. Neither husband nor wife knows in advance how the other will behave as a parent responsible for rearing a dependent child. Sometimes the behavior that emerges is upsetting because it reveals new and unsuspected characteristics in a spouse. Many unconscious ideas emerge when a baby is born. For example, all of a sudden you may find your spouse acting like your mother-in-law or father-in-law, and you don't like it. You never objected to your in-laws' behavior, perhaps because they were not sufficiently a part of your life to become objectionable. But your spouse is. When he patterns his behavior after the parent he usually identifies with, you get annoyed. Likewise, some people have unresolved ideas and conflicting emotions about their own parents even though they are adult and married. When the spouse of an individual like this becomes a parent, this type of individual reacts toward his spouse not as a spouse but as a parent. And this person's unresolved conflicts with his own parents significantly affects how he behaves toward his spouse.

One new mother I advised had never been able to make even small decisions without consulting her own mother. She described her father as being very passive, told me that her mother had always made the decisions for him, and said how much he resented it. Then she went on to say that she still feels the need to ask her mother to come along whenever she shops. Otherwise, she can't decide what to buy. In fact, she had just left her mother before coming to see me. (She proudly showed me the new sweater that both of them had decided on.) As she elaborated on her relationship with her mother, it became clear that she resents her mother for her dependency, which has extended into her child-rearing functions. What is even more significant is that she all of a sudden finds herself making unreasonable demands on her own husband and tends to negate whatever he decides. She claims that she can't understand her compulsion to reject all her husband's decisions about caring for their new baby, even though she still needs her own mother to decide what sweater she will buy. Clearly, this woman has identified with her own mother and consequently treats her husband the way her mother treats her father. Since she now has a baby of her own, she tends more than ever to treat her husband the way her father was treated. To say the least, psychological factors like this can stress a marriage when a child is born. If problems like these persist, professional help should be sought to prevent the problem from snowballing into serious difficulty.

I don't mean to de-emphasize the pleasures of having a new baby at home, but when you are prepared for a situation in advance, you are more effective in coping with it. It will make things easier if both parents share the responsibility of rearing children. I cannot emphasize too much that if one parent can take over for the other, it minimizes the fatigue and the amount of time each parent has to contribute. Both parents end up benefiting. So does your child. Attempts to cut corners or turn over all these responsibilities to others can later lead to serious emotional difficulties that will drain vast amounts of your time, financial resources, and emotional resources. Preventing trouble is always easier than repairing the damage.

- X -

Meeting Your Child's Emotional Needs

The impact of early experience on later behavior is heavily documented in scientific studies. Emotional stability during adolescence and adulthood has been proved over and over again to be significantly influenced by what happens during the very first years of life. When an individual suffers from an abnormal emotional problem, the doctor involved takes a detailed history of the patient's early experiences in order to locate the events that unbalanced that person's later behavioral adjustment. At the popular level, when acts of violence—murders, assassination attempts, skyjackings—are committed, the news media invariably investigate the criminal's early life experiences. Reporters go to his home town and interview teachers, parents, and neighbors.

Most people instinctively know about the importance of early life, and practically all theories of personality development acknowledge its significance. Nevertheless, society has done little to prevent emotional disturbances from taking root in our children. The time it later takes to treat adults with emotional problems and the cost of that treatment is astronomical in relation to the results that are achieved. It would be far easier, cheaper, and more humane to prevent these problems in the first place.

In the years I spent working with adults who had emotional problems, I was increasingly impressed by the relationship between my patients' disturbed early lives and the severity of their later mental problems. This led me to my present work with children, where I have a better opportunity to prevent the development of serious emotional problems, frequently by educating parents. Most parents keenly want to do what is best for their child, and, clearly, parents can have great influence on their children's early development. Despite their good intentions, the number of well-meaning, emotionally well-adjusted parents whose children eventually develop emotional problems always impresses me. Over and over again in my professional work with emotionally disturbed children, I have said to myself, "If only I could have gotten to the parents of that child! I could probably have prevented the problem from developing in the first place." It seems ironic that the people who have the greatest impact on the development of the human beings who are their children have so little training about human behavior. Of course, it is only fair to say that some of the emotional problems that I have encountered in my practice developed because parents followed bad recommendations. Pediatricians and other health professionals too frequently give advice that either is based on foolish myths or is totally refuted by clinical and scientific observations. For example, as we have seen, lots of parents have been told, "Do not pick up your baby when it cries. You will spoil it." "If you pick up your baby whenever it cries, your baby will always want to be picked up." "If you pick up your baby whenever it cries, you are neurotic." "You shouldn't pick up your baby when it cries because crying is good for the lungs." Of course, all of these statements are untrue, and acting upon them can only be detrimental to your child's emotional health. Meeting the emotional needs of your baby during the first year of his life is no small task. It requires a great deal of time and patience. It also requires that you learn to see the world through your child's eyes, and you must be able to recognize the meaning of your child's behavior. At the same time, it will be helpful to acknowledge your own natural inclination to respond to your baby's needs.

Many people have been led to believe that a newborn baby is something of a vegetable. She is supposed to have few differentiated responses, and she is supposed to be incapable of responding. That's just not so. When your baby is born, she is capable of seeing, hearing, feeling, tasting, smelling, and sensing movement. In fact, your baby has a strong need to use her senses. If she does not, usually because she is cared for in a way that does not permit stimulation of her senses, she may become bored. Boredom, as most of us know, can be a most unpleasant and uncomfortable emotional state. When babies get bored, they generally cry until somebody does something to alleviate the boredom. This fact, which has been scientifically examined, becomes clear to parents when they find that picking up a baby who appears physically comfortable causes the baby to stop crying.

It is quite true that babies who receive stimulation, usually by being picked up and moved about, seem to want more stimulation and, therefore, want to be picked up more often. To me this is a marvelous phenomenon which indicates that your child enjoys stimulation that centers around people and, particularly, that he is happy being around you. While it may sometimes seem a burden to meet his need for sensory stimulation, providing that stimulation diligently will pay dividends over and over again later in life. As your baby grows up, you will find that as his physical capabilities increase so will his interest in learning about his environment. He will develop the kind of healthy curiosity that helps him explore and understand the world. Obviously, a child who is anxious to learn

about the world will eventually have more resources to draw upon than a child raised in a
restrictive environment that lacked sufficient
stimulation. Babies who receive inadequate
stimulation frequently become distrustful,
thwarted, and unhappy. They tend to withdraw
from people and become apprehensive about
newness. They often show fretful, clinging behavior for long periods of time. Incidentally, the
kind of stimulation your baby needs is the kind
that you provide by holding him, cuddling him,
and playing with him the way you spontaneously do in the course of everyday life. It is not
necessary to embark upon a formally planned
set of activities organized in modules by colleagues of mine whose findings in the behavioral laboratory are packaged and put in programs which are supposed to promote learning
during early infancy. I dislike these kinds of programs because they generally interfere with the
spontaneity of your relationship with your child.
His learning will take place naturally as he satisfies his innate curiosity.

It is instructive to examine more closely the
way a baby does learn. All you have to do at first
is let your baby watch you carefully. Believe me,
she will be sensitive to the way you react to what
she does. When she smears carrots all over your
face and you become angry, she will know you're
angry. Then she will try it again, not to make you
more angry, but to see if her behavior will cause
you to have the same reaction. Don't be surprised that your baby smiles when you get angry

the second time. Her smile does not mean that she is pleased about your annoyance. It does mean that your child has solved a puzzle and now knows what makes you angry. She also knows she can elicit a given response under given circumstances. In fact, your baby's behavior is not unlike that of a research scientist testing a hypothesis. A scientist conducts an investigation, and when she comes up with findings, she repeats the study to see if the findings are valid—that is, to see if she gets the same results the second time around. Most scientists react with a feeling of exhilaration similar to your baby's when they have validated a hypothesis. Then they publish their findings in a scientific journal. Obviously, your baby will not publish her findings, so if you are not alert, you may not be aware of what she has learned.

Since your baby has had very little experience in this world, he will learn from each situation that he encounters, and he will record what he learns in his brain to use later on when he needs it. You will have to be consistent in your reactions if your baby is to learn easily. If you laugh when he smears carrots on your face the first time, and then scowl and get angry the second time, your child will have to test his hypothesis many, many more times than if your reaction was consistent both the first and second time. In fact, it generally confuses a child when a parent reacts inconsistently. To find out what he wants to know, the child will have to test his hypothesis repeatedly, and periodically, in an attempt to find consistency. If you do happen to be inconsistent, and you're bound to sometimes, your child's repeated testing of your reaction may make you feel that your child is out to get you and make your life miserable. From your point of view your reaction is reasonable. Actually, your child is simply trying to find out exactly what makes the world work. Sometime during the second part of the first year of life, your child will begin testing the same hypothesis on different people. He is trying to find out if the way you react is the way the rest of the world reacts. Incidentally, although it is important for you to be consistent, it is not necessary that the whole world be consistent. If other people's reactions do not match yours, your child will learn that people are individuals and have different responses to the same situation.

During the first year of life, providing stimulation for your baby is terribly important, and so is fostering dependency. In fact, your baby should positively enjoy his dependency and find total security within his dependency relationship with you. Nature has organized human behavioral development in such a way that any human being goes through a long period of dependency early in life. A baby does require extended parental care. In fact, if the child is to survive, his parents are almost forced to be close to him during the first few years of life. The way nature planned it causes your child to become very attached to you during his dependent first year of life, and it is precisely this attachment that affords you the opportunity to develop his emotional security, teach trust in people, and build his sense of self-esteem. Later on you can use these three qualities to teach him a sense of discipline and, ultimately, to instill the capacity to make judgments about what is right and wrong. I cannot emphasize this point enough. Establishing emotional security during the first year of life when your baby's normal, natural dependency is there for you to use is crucial to your child's later sense of self-esteem, his capacity to cope with rules and regulations, and, ultimately, his ability to develop a conscience. True, some professionals advocate that you should not allow your baby to become too attached to you or dependent on you because they feel that you will be tied down to your child. You will be tied down, but if your baby does not have the opportunity to be dependent upon you, it will interfere with your baby's learning the skills of independence. I believe it is perfectly appropriate for your baby to be dependent during the first year of life, and again, I urge you to treat your baby accordingly. For only through being first dependent can a child ultimately achieve independence. After all, if one is not dependent to begin with, how can one become independent?

Satisfaction in the dependent relationship with her parents also helps a baby learn to relate deeply on a one-to-one basis. A child who is prevented early in life from establishing a deep-rooted dependency relationship with some one person, perhaps because she has been taken care of by numerous people, often has difficulty establishing deep, personal relationships in adulthood. Studies of infants and young children who live in institutions, and necessarily relate to many people without close contact with any one individual, show this point to be true. Children brought up under these circumstances are well known to have defects in their capacity to relate meaningfully to other individuals. Since they constantly have to be prepared to learn to know still another person, they find it difficult if not impossible to get really involved with anyone. Sometimes they tend to cling to whoever happens to be around, and they show little discrimination about people. They often approach anyone available for whatever kind of emotional support the other person will give them.

/ If during the first year of life a baby's dependency need and his need for sensory stimulation are met, he will begin to show an increased desire to do things by himself. He quickly learns, usually before he is a year old, the sense of satisfaction that comes from using his own resources to move around in his environment and manipulate objects. These elements of independence emerge readily if a child's early infantile needs were satisfied. Since I always respect nature's way of accomplishing things, I cannot help noting that your baby's need for stimulation and his expression of his dependence frequently occur at the same time: namely, when he begins to cry!

Too many people interpret a baby's cry as a selfish demand for attention. They take it as a personal insult when a baby cries. I say your baby should not be abandoned when he is crying, even if all your attempts to comfort him seem futile. It is far better to hold your baby in your arms while he is uncomfortable than to abandon him behind a closed door. "Colicky" babies are sometimes uncomfortable for many months. If their parents elect to hold them, even though they cannot seem to relieve the babies' discomfort, when the colic subsides for reasons of its own, the babies then behave as if they had been happy all their lives. They act like other babies who did not happen to have the misfortune to experience a lot of unpleasant abdominal pain.

Many babies show healthy emotional development until parents decide to let a baby "cry it out." The next time she cries, the baby is allowed to cry until she stops. Then the baby seems to give up crying, which initially pleases the parents. Often these babies are described by their parents as "good babies," meaning that they are compliant and place few demands upon their parents—until their emotionally disturbed reactions begin to show up later on. Then the parents realize that their child not only gave up crying, but gave up looking other people straight in the face, playing appropriately with toys, and relating appropriately to other people.

I was recently asked to evaluate a ten-month-old child to determine why there had been a sudden change in his behavior. Apparently, he acted normally until he was eight months of age. He smiled and babbled, recognized his mother and father, and showed normal apprehension toward strangers. He played with toys, crumpled paper, sat erect, crawled around, and pulled himself up to a standing position. In general, he was a happy baby with a vigorous curiosity. When he was in his playpen he cried to get out so that he could explore the world. At night time he seemed a bit fretful, but whenever his mother or father held him, he seemed able to relax and go to sleep. From their description of his crying and general discomfort, it sounded to me as if he were in some pain from teething. These parents discussed their baby's crying with friends, their pediatrician, and a cousin who was majoring in psychology. They all advised them to let the baby cry it out. "Put him to bed, close the door, turn up the music on your radio. Eventually he will stop crying and go to sleep." Instinctively they felt it would be wrong to let their baby cry unattended and they fought within themselves against doing it. Finally they succumbed to the others' opinions. They let their baby cry it out for five successive nights. Each night the length of crying did decrease from one half hour the first night to five minutes the fourth night. "We conquered our anxiety," these parents told me, "and it worked. Our baby went to sleep easily. He became a 'good baby,' placed few demands on us, and spent hours by himself whenever we left him."

Upon further inquiry, I learned that the baby's curiosity soon decreased; he frequently played by himself, sometimes rocking back and forth and sometimes passing his hands in front of his face in a rhythmical way. He tended to arch his back away from his parents when he was picked up, and he showed considerably less eye-to-eye contact with them. He no longer pulled himself up to the standing position and spent considerably more time on his back. He even needed to be awakened to be fed and seemed totally disinterested in his environment. These parents, who had succeeded in transforming a curious baby into a "good baby," began to be alarmed only when this "good" behavior coincided with an arrest in the child's development.

I saw this youngster after all the specialists ruled out a physical disorder. The neurologist found him normal. So did the endocrinologist, the expert in genetic disorders and birth defects, and all the other specialists who evaluated him before me. Their diagnosis was "psychomotor retardation of unknown origin." I agreed, it was psychomotor retardation, but the origin seemed no mystery. The arrested psychomotor development coincided with his being ignored by his parents when he needed help. He learned what he was taught and tuned out the world. In a sense, he was forced to give up his curiosity and his will to develop. He had complied with his parents' wishes: They had reacted as if he didn't exist and he had learned to react similarly—as if he, in fact, didn't exist for them. He is in his own world—tuned out. While this does not always happen to all babies who are allowed to cry for long periods of time, it happens to enough of them to make me think that it is too risky to let your baby cry it out.

No matter how difficult it may be for you to meet the emotional needs of your baby during the first year of life, it is indeed a worthwhile investment. The more responsive you are to your baby's infantile needs, the sooner your baby will be able to give up these needs and move on to more mature stages in development. In my clinical experience, I cannot tell you how many times I have seen children suffer from the disinterest of parents who were too busy to heed their children's emotional requirements. Ironically, in the long run, these same children force their parents to spend even more of their time to repair the damage caused by their earlier neglect. The way human development works makes it impossible to give your baby later on in life what he should have gotten during those critical early months. Once the appropriate time has passed and your child's needs are not met, you absolutely cannot reverse time and undo the effects of his loss.

-XI-

Organizing a Life of Your Own Away from Your Baby

I know you cannot live your entire life centered around your child, and I realize you cannot stay with your baby every minute of every day. Nevertheless, I think you should know what being separated from you means to a little baby. Then you can arrange to get away when you need to and, at the same time, provide for your baby's emotional needs. Studies show that if a baby is separated from his parents for long periods of time, he or she may begin not to respond to them. That reaction is his primitive form of protest. If you persist in creating separations, particularly in times of stress, your baby may develop a kind of emotional detachment. When this happens, some parents feel they have taught their babies not to miss them when they go away. But what the baby has actually learned is that his parents are not there when he needs them. During the first two years of life, even short periods of separation can cause a baby to react this way. Upset parents have reported to me over and over again that their babies tended to ignore them after they had been away on a trip lasting only two or three days. In that short a time, your child does become attached to the person you have left to care for him during your absence and that new attachment can make your baby turn to the other person rather than to you for comfort and help.

It is hard to set exact guidelines for how long a period of time it is safe for you to be away from your child how soon in his life. Perhaps we should take notice of the guidelines of nature. People who breast feed their babies are necessarily brought into close contact with them frequently, at intervals of no less than three to four hours at a time. While the baby is fed, the parent also insures that the baby's needs for contact and closeness are being met. This may be one way of measuring the maximum separation you should create between you and your infant. In short, if you have to be away from your baby—and I know you will have to from time to time—make it for several short intervals rather than one long one.

I think it is a good idea to enlist the assistance of baby-sitters soon after you come home from the hospital. They will give you your chance to get away from your baby now and then to tend to other matters, and they will also get your baby used to being handled by others from time to time. It usually works best to have perhaps two or three baby-sitters that you call upon occasionally, but make sure that all of them are responsive to your baby's emotional needs in a way that is consistent with your philosophy of child rearing. Any baby-sitter should like children, enjoy playing with them, and have a sincere feeling of warmth that is expressed spontaneously in his or her handling of your child. If you do not feel comfortable with a particular baby-sitter, do not hesitate to send that person away. You must, absolutely must, feel comfortable with the baby-sitter who is caring for your child. I, myself, am more impressed by baby-sitters who show a sincere interest in making a child happy than I am by a baby-sitter who, however experienced, appears overly concerned with neatness and cleanliness. And I particularly dislike baby-sitters who ignore your wishes and instructions, as they send you off from your own home saying, "Don't be nervous. I know what I'm doing, so you have nothing to worry about." At first you may find it difficult to leave anyone else in charge of your child, which is a perfectly normal and natural feeling to have. In fact, some people choose never to have baby-sitters. They take their children with them everywhere. While I have no theoretical objections to this approach, if you are forced to be away from your child later on for one reason or another, your baby will then have a difficult time suddenly adjusting to another person's caring for him. For this reason, it is probably wiser to find and use a few baby-sitters that both you and your baby feel comfortable with.

Whenever a baby-sitter comes to your home, you ought to arrange things in a manner that allows enough time to let your baby become familiar with the baby-sitter before you leave. Generally speaking, this takes between a half an hour and an hour. The exact amount of time varies with the age and temperament of your child and also with his familiarity with the baby-sitter. Even though newborn babies apparently show little awareness of strangers, it is still important to have the baby-sitter come early so that there is no chance that your baby will be apprehensive. Incidentally, you should also arrange for the sitter to come while your child is awake. I cannot tell you how many times I have seen sleep disturbances develop because a baby wakes up to find a stranger caring for her after she was put down to sleep by her parents. Understandably this shocking surprise may cause your baby to cry in the hope that her cry will bring forth her parent. When her cries do not produce the expected parent, a child can become panic-stricken. She may then begin to be apprehensive about going to sleep at any time or letting you out of her sight. In the child's mind, going to sleep has become the equivalent of making you go away. So under no circumstances should you sneak away when you are going out. It is far better for your child to be aware of your leaving, even if she cries, than it is for you to hide your going to prevent her from crying. You will only create far more stress that just might have very bad long-term effects.

Having a steady parade of different baby-sitters, none of whom is particularly familiar to your child, can cause your child to become apprehensive about strangers. She begins to associate a stranger with a separation from her parents. Since she doesn't like the separation, she doesn't like the stranger. And making frequent changes can have more serious effects. In my professional practice, I frequently encounter serious emotional problems in children who have had lots of different people caring for them. The child is thus prevented from ever establishing a continuing relationship with any adult, particularly if the parents themselves are never around because they prefer to let other people care for their children. Children who are treated this way are deprived not only of interested, concerned parents whose children are important to them, but of the chance for a consistent, parent-like relationship with some other person.

When parents ask me how old a baby should be before they go off alone on a vacation, I usually answer by asking, "Why can't you take your child with you?" Vacationing together is the ideal arrangement for your child. It invariably involves more work for you, but I think that's one of the responsibilities of parenthood. Sometimes it can be arranged conveniently by taking along the person with whom you would have left your child. You have the assistance you need to let you have some time to yourselves, and yet you are still close to your child. Consequently, he will not experience the feeling of abandonment or desertion that often leads to fretfulness, excessive clinging, and sleep problems. I know many people would like to be able to get away from young children totally for a week or two, and although I would like to assure you that this practice will cause no bad effects, I cannot. In actual fact, it is more likely that on your return your child will ignore you, or perhaps have regressed in his behavior. He may even have been depressed and refused to eat while you were gone. These are the normal, understandable reactions of a baby who truly wants and needs his parents. Ideally, you should wait to take trips away from your baby until he can talk and understands time well enough for you to explain "now," "later," "tomorrow," and "the day after." This generally becomes possible when your child is close to three years old.

I see nothing at all that will be harmful to your baby if you take him on vacation trips. Your child will become accustomed to new places and new situations in the sheltering presence of his parents who provide the security he needs to adjust to new environments. If you do travel with little children, try to find out in advance if children are readily accommodated where you are going. If you are going on a plane, particularly if you are going on a long flight, it is generally a good idea to inform the airline that you will be taking a baby aboard. In many instances, special treatment is provided that makes your trip easier. Incidentally, when aircraft take off and pressurization takes place, you have learned that swallowing or opening your mouth causes unpleasant sensations in your ears to go away. Babies do not know these tricks, but you can help them by giving them something to suck on while the plane is changing altitudes. When a baby screams on an airplane, most people think that the baby is afraid of the takeoff or landing. The explanation is more probably that the change in pressure caused severe pain in the baby's ears.

Many parents wonder about the advisability of taking little babies to restaurants. I see no reason why they should not, even at night. Having your baby along may force you to put aside your meal long enough to tend to his needs from time to time, but nothing in the process harms your baby. And from a practical point of view, taking a baby to a restaurant enables you to get out once in a while without incurring the additional expense of a baby-sitter. Obviously, you would want to steer clear of very formal places, where the emphasis is on anything but the needs of little babies. One word of caution: Prepare yourself for some disapproving soul telling you that you are interfering with your baby's need for sleep or that "Night air is bad for your child." Like much other advice, this platitude has no basis whatsoever! I defy anyone to differentiate a jar of night air from a jar of daylight air.

One matter of great concern to all parents, veterans as well as new parents, is their privacy:

how to achieve it and how to maintain it. When children are little and cannot get around on their own, it is relatively easy for parents to maintain their privacy, particularly the privacy necessary to engage in sexual intercourse. Most people know that it is psychologically best for children not to be present while their parents are engaging in sexual activity, even if the children are tiny and do not understand what is going on. The physical actions of the parents and the sounds they make can easily be misunderstood by a little child, who will think his parents are actively fighting. If by chance your infant or baby has been present while you had intercourse, I do not think it will necessarily damage him forever. But I would try not to repeat the experience. Actually, from your own point of view, the presence of a child can only serve to inhibit what should be spontaneous.

Perhaps the best way to protect your privacy is to establish some rules right at the start. When your child is old enough to turn a door knob, you should make the rule that when a door is shut, no one—including you as a parent—opens that door without knocking first. If it becomes commonplace for doors to be shut and then knocked upon before being opened, things will be better for everyone. Because children are very curious, if you close the door only when you are having intercourse, your child will quickly learn that something forbidden is going on. The closed door will imply that you have restricted your child, which will probably intensify his curiosity about what's happening inside. It's much better to have taught him about privacy as a matter of course. Actually you might as well realize that even though it shouldn't happen, eventually your child will, sooner or later, inadvertently and momentarily interrupt this most private of all times.

Although privacy for sexual intercourse seems appropriate, I see nothing wrong whatsoever in appearing nude before your children, who should become familiar with the human body, the differences between males and females, and the changes that occur in the body as a person matures. If parents constantly hide themselves from their child and worry lest he see their "private parts," the child soon begins to wonder what his parents are hiding that is so wonderful and valuable. Little children have very productive imaginations and distort all sorts of things in very elaborate ways. Many children whose curiosity about the human body has been heightened by overdone parental modesty are often disappointed when they find out what other people's bodies are actually like. Sometimes, extreme parental modesty leads a child to develop a compulsion to see naked people. Peeping Toms and voyeurs act this way. If you want to avoid distorting your child's natural curiosity into compulsive behavior, act casually and matter-of-factly about nudity. Don't, of course, sexually stimulate your children. Also, bear in mind that when a little child stands before you her eye level view straight ahead is of your genitals.

Thus, she may get the idea that things are bigger than they are. Hopefully you will make your child feel free to talk about his or her own body with you and ask you questions about yours. Discussing matters like these openly helps your child understand one part of life more fully and avoids making certain subjects taboo. Any child needs help to come to terms with his or her own sexuality as he or she progresses through the various stages in development. By being casual about nudity now you are making yourself a more askable person about sexual matters later on.

Many new parents are concerned whether or not it is good for a child if both his parents work. In order to answer this question effectively, I have to make my position about men and women working clear. I am absolutely in favor of both men and women preparing themselves for and undertaking some sort of vocation. At the same time, I believe that young people should be taught what's involved in parenthood so they know all about the demands that parenthood will place upon them. If the educational process is successful, young people should be free to choose whether or not to have children. They ought to be able to choose freely, and they should not feel the pressure of the old social stigma that not having children is selfish or immature. I myself see absolutely nothing wrong with deciding to be childless. Growing up and slipping passively into parenthood causes too many problems. If young people, particularly young women, are educated in a way that gives them alternatives to parenthood, then, and only then, is it possible for them to elect to be parents in a positive rather than a passive way. However, if a person does decide to become a parent, I think that positive decision includes a commitment to meet the physical and emotional needs of the child he plans to bring into this world. In my view, having a child and turning him over to others for upbringing is irresponsible unless there are absolutely no other alternatives available. We as a society have been inclined to downgrade parenthood, and this, I think, has sometimes led people to view parenthood as a hobby or part-time occupation. It's just not so.

Once you or anyone else has decided to become a parent, I think you should put the needs of your child first, particularly during the first three years of his life. Some professionals in my field take the position that parents come first. They believe the happy parent is the best parent. If happiness means being away from your child and hiring someone to take care of her while you are doing whatever makes you happy, so be it. They say your child will benefit in the long run. I absolutely do not agree. Any child wants to be important in her parents' lives. If a child, particularly during the early formative years, begins to feel that she is less important to her parents than some other things, this feeling of inferiority interferes with the development of her all-important sense of self-esteem. This is why I generally suggest that if it is not absolutely necessary for both parents to work, one parent should not work during the first nine, ten, or eleven months of the baby's life. That time should be fully devoted to parenthood.

If the period of time that both parents are away at their jobs does not exceed three or four hours, a child will not necessarily feel a sense of neglect or loss of self-esteem if both his parents are working. However, if both parents work, either the father or mother should plan to go home to be with the child in the middle of the day for perhaps two to three hours. Since children under three still need a great deal of parental attention, the parent should use that block of time to be with his child and attend to family needs. This arrangement is far better than custodial care. I find the individual time and attention necessary during this stage of a young child's development rarely comes about when a child is cared for with a group of others. Employers really ought to make it possible for parents of children under the age of three to organize their schedules to consider the needs of their children. Too often the rigidity of our working environments makes it impossible to be both a happy employee and a good parent, though an individual could be both. Incidentally, in some cultures, the life-style simplifies this problem. The siesta common in Latin countries brings families together in the middle of the day.

When a child is three years old he requires much less parental time and attention. He is ready to attend school for half a day. A parent will have more time to work, but it is still important that a young child who attends school have a parent waiting to greet him when he returns from school. I know many adults who describe in detail their memories of coming home to an empty house. Significantly, they also remember feeling unimportant, neglected, and angry with their parents, who could never seem to be there.

As an advocate of the interests of children, and one who is deeply concerned with gratifying infantile needs to prevent the development of serious emotional problems later on, I have often been misunderstood as one who believes mothers should not work. I have no objections whatsoever to working mothers or, for that matter, to working fathers provided that the little children they have chosen to bring into this world do not suffer. If parents are too committed to their work or professional life to satisfy their children's needs, I think it would be better for all of us if these people did not have children in the first place. And it might well be better for the parents themselves. As any child attempts to adjust to the world, he soon learns how to satisfy his needs in the most efficient and economical way. A child whose working parents treat him with benign neglect soon learns the best way to demand their interest. If he is paid attention to only when he is ill, he soon uses physical complaints to get his busy parents' recognition. Sometimes being destructive does the trick, or getting into trouble at school.

Recently, I kept an appointment with a five-

year-old boy and his parents. They had been referred to me by the principal of the school where
the child attended kindergarten. Apparently the
boy stole and engaged in other kinds of disruptive behavior. My secretary reported that she
had had a difficult time arranging an appointment because both parents worked. The child's
mother made it clear that she would not neglect
her work as a stockbroker. Yet, when we finally
worked out a time at her convenience, her husband, an attorney, said he could not make it.
Thus, I found myself in the very significant but
rather unfortunate position of having to choose
between denying them an appointment or rearranging my own schedule, which would be a
great inconvenience. I chose the latter course,
partly out of my desire to assist this youngster
who needed help but also to validate my initial
impression that the problems we were having
arranging an appointment were also the reasons
for the child's behavior.

When the boy and his parents came to my
office I learned that this child had been unplanned. His parents had never given a thought
to parenthood, and his mother confessed that
she went through with her pregnancy with the
intention of hiring someone to raise her child for
her. Both parents were obviously people who assumed the responsibilities they undertook. Unfortunately, they did not view their child as a
responsibility but as something that sort of came
along and happened. Moreover, both parents admitted openly that neither one had much pa-

tience for or interest in the activities children enjoy.

After getting this brief picture of the parents' attitudes and a glimpse of the psychological environment in which their son lived, I focused on his disruptive behavior in school and his stealing. He apparently caused difficulties for his teacher by deliberately drawing on other children's pictures, adding things to other children's block constructions, and giving other children cookies and juice after the teacher cleared things up at the end of snack time. My impression was that the boy needed to express himself and be meaningful to other people but felt unimportant or inadequate. It seemed he was unable to rely on his own abilities, as if he lacked a sense of self-esteem. Incidentally, as his parents described his stealing, it became clear that their greatest concern was their own embarrassment rather than their son's disturbed behavior. When I urged them to elaborate further on their son's stealing, they told me that after he stole, he generally withheld the object just long enough for everyone in the class to search for it. He then produced it as if he had found it himself. The first few times this happened no one mentioned it, but after it became a pattern, the teacher wondered what the boy was trying to communicate through his behavior. The teacher was obviously sensitive to the child's problems and telephoned his parents to suggest professional consultation.

After speaking with this youngster, it seemed clear that he needed to feel important to

167

people and that he was obviously not getting that need satisfied in his relationship with his parents. Equally obviously, he was neither a crook nor a criminal. He only "stole" objects such as pieces of puzzles, which placed him in the position of being absolutely essential before some games could be complete. What he was doing was not really stealing but making it possible to find things other people were looking for. He was trying to gain recognition. By finding the puzzle piece or other object that was lost, he was indeed making himself important. For that moment, at least, he was a hero.

When I explained the meaning of this child's behavior to his parents, their reaction was, "What can we do about it? We both work and have no time. After all, our work is extremely important." While it might have been better for everyone involved if these people had not had a child in the first place, I couldn't see any value in saying so. I simply acknowledged to myself that these parents were among the many productive people engaging in useful work who gave little or no thought to the responsibility they fell into. Like many others, they convincingly told me that everyone ought to know what parenthood is about—before they become parents.

-XII-

When and How to Discipline

One of the great concerns of new parents, and, for that matter, of all parents, is discipline. When should discipline begin? How should it be instituted? Will it harm a child? Won't it interfere with the expression of a child's natural feeling? Who should handle discipline? The answers to these questions and many more like them require an understanding of what discipline is. To begin with, I would like to make it clear that disciplining a child basically means teaching him to act voluntarily according to a set of rules and regulations that define what is acceptable and what is unacceptable behavior. The word discipline is commonly used interchangeably with the word punishment. They are not, however, interchangeable; punishment, in my terminology, is the price or the penalty a child pays for violating the rules and regulations that are established as the basis of discipline.

Parents are sometimes surprised when I tell them that children actually like discipline, even enjoy it, because they feel more secure and protected when their parents set rules and regulations and enforce them consistently. All children enjoy games because they absolutely adore the idea of engaging in an activity that has pattern and predictability. They are alternately amused and challenged by a controlled situation. They constantly try to find out exactly what the rules and regulations of the game are, or in more general terms, what principles are involved. Many times I have observed a group of three- or four-year-old children left to play in a room. Within minutes, they organize activities that have rules and regulations. In a sense, they start a game which is one method of finding out about each other by interacting in a predictable way. In the game of life itself, children search for life's rules and regulations as a way of enhancing communication. They constantly test the world, exploring what makes things happen, if they happen consistently, and whether they happen the same way under different circumstances. A child whose parents have taught her the rules and regulations of acceptable behavior in our society understands discipline. Put another way, discipline is a form of language—a behavioral communication that a child must understand and master in order to live happily among other people. Fortunately, children like the discipline of a game. It comes naturally, and so it can be with discipline in general.

Children are best disciplined by parents, especially parents who love them and are trusted by them. Parents who spent little time with their children or who provided little satisfaction of their needs early in life are not as effective in setting rules and regulations later on. After all, why should a child care about her parents' reactions if they have never shown any particular concern about the child's needs? If parents have satisfied a child's early needs and minimized her frustrations, she will feel secure in the presence of her parents and will trust them to protect her. This kind of child will be inclined to allow her parents to interpret the demands the outside world will make on her behavior. She trusts her parents when they say something has to be done this way and not that way. Generally speaking, children show the greatest response to those people they love. That's why the key tool for parents in establishing discipline is their own reaction to a child's behavior. Expressing pleasure and pride in, and acceptance of, behavior that is approved reinforces that behavior. On the other hand, expressing annoyance, dissatisfaction, and rejection of behavior that is disapproved makes it clear to a child that he should not behave in that fashion. If a parent disciplines by expressing his satisfaction or displeasure, it helps a child understand that his behavior is central to the emotional reactions of others. Giving a child a present as a reward for acceptable behavior and taking things away as punishment simply places the emphasis on the material objects and not on his behavior. Furthermore, it makes an object more important than it should be if it is taken away as a punishment.

Instituting discipline is a continuation of your concern and love for your child that was originally expressed by meeting all his needs when he was totally dependent on you. It is a method of enhancing your growing child's developing sense of self-esteem while protecting him from danger and teaching him how to act in a socially acceptable fashion. It is a special way of showing that you care and are concerned for the welfare of your child, and it is a method of showing him how to cope acceptably with his curiosity in the world. Discipline teaches that it is only through learning to accept limitations that one can understand the concept of freedom. After all, how could one possibly learn about freedom without understanding limitations? It would be similar to understanding what the word "yes" means if the very language does not include the word "no."

A child will periodically test out the rules and regulations you set as part of discipline. For this reason you must be consistent. Similarly, you must enforce whatever punishment you have established for violation of the rules. Threatening a child with a punishment and not carrying it out weakens your position, makes your child anxious that you do not care about her behavior, and intensifies her need to be certain that you mean what you say. When you do punish a child, you should fit the punishment to the crime. Take care not to be too severe. Mild punishments are more effective in the long run. Severe punishment is not only cruel but will not work. Your child will only feel that you have hurt him and will not learn that the behavior that caused him to be punished was wrong. Severe punishment can even lead a child to feel that you are wrong, not he. Always warn a child in advance what the punishment will be if he violates the rules. If you do, your child will know you are not unfair when he gets punished and will learn that he can make a conscious choice about the way he is going to behave and the results of that behavior.

Punishing infants and babies is extremely difficult. They can understand your approval and disapproval of what they are doing, but it is almost impossible to warn a ten-month-old in advance. When your baby's behavior is placing him in clear physical danger, as when he is climbing up on window sills near open second-story windows, I think in such cases a mild spanking is appropriate while you express your intense disapproval. The spanking may traumatize your child somewhat, but I would rather have a living traumatized child than a well-adjusted one lying on the ground underneath the window.

I know many parents believe that anything

a child does willfully should be accepted as an important expression of feeling. They think that any attempt to limit a child's freedom of expression will only cause frustration, repressions, and possibly neuroses. I do not agree. In fact, I believe the exact opposite. Everyone has to learn to channel her feelings and actions in a socially useful way. To do so requires learning to accept some frustration and learning to overcome frustration in a way that does not infringe upon the rights of others. It is not psychologically healthy for a child to pick up a jar of strawberry jam, throw it across the room, and watch it smash against the wall as his parent sits passively by, excusing this activity as creative and useful. His parent's inaction gives the child a false impression of what society will regard as acceptable behavior. I wouldn't feel comfortable having a jam-throwing child in my home, and I doubt that you would either. So the parent who thinks he is helping his child be free may actually be limiting his child's freedom, since most people prefer to keep a healthy distance between themselves and a destructive child.

The time to begin disciplining is when your child begins to move around in his environment and carry out voluntary and controlled actions, usually as he's getting to be a year old. As your child begins to show a capacity to drop things, throw things, tear things, or crawl from one place to another, to that degree your child is ready for discipline. Setting and enforcing rules and regulations before your child is capable of doing any of these things is meaningless. It can only confuse and overwhelmingly frustrate any child. Obviously, the rules and regulations you establish and enforce when your child begins to need discipline should be set at a level that your child can comprehend. Thus, while it is quite possible to teach an eight- or nine-month-old that it is all right to tear newspapers but not magazines, it is not possible to teach her that she can tear yesterday's paper, but not today's. Since she has not learned to read words or recognize dates, that would be too much to expect.

If you are surprised that a child less than a year old can be disciplined not to tear magazines, while she is allowed to destroy newspapers, let me explain how it's done. Allow your child to approach a coffee table piled with magazines and newspapers. She will begin to play with them and will look at you as she explores the piles to discover your reaction. As she begins to tear a magazine, take it away, say "No" very firmly, and be emphatic in expressing your annoyance so that your displeasure is clearly understood. Simply murmuring "no" while smiling at a young child will probably not register. Although you must make your dissatisfaction absolutely clear, do not act so displeased that your child stops understanding your displeasure and starts becoming afraid. Now give the magazine back to your child. More than likely, if she has not been frightened into stopping her efforts to learn, she will make another attempt to tear the magazine, and you should again react in exactly the same way. Then your child will begin to see the consistent pattern in your behavior. She will probably go on to repeat her action several times in varying ways to establish clearly that you are indeed reacting to what she is doing and that you really mean what you say. Actually, she thinks all this is sort of like a game! To make your point absolutely clear, somewhere along the line you can pick up a newspaper, tear it and then show your child that she may tear the newspaper. After your child has torn the newspaper, she may again try to tear the magazine. You will have to express your displeasure yet again if the magazine is about to be torn. Your child may have to repeat the experiment involving the newspaper and the magazine a number of times before she learns exactly what the rules and regulations that govern this particular behavior are. If you are going to teach her, that is, discipline her, not to tear magazines, you will have to allow a lot of time and be very patient if she is to learn all of what you want her to understand.

Let me give you another example involving a very common occurrence. Your child is sitting in a high chair holding a cup of milk in his hand. For no particular reason your child happens to twist his wrist. He finds to his fascination that when he twists his wrist, it makes the milk leave his cup and fall to the floor. Then he notices that he has changed the color of the floor from green to white! And he is even more fascinated to observe that his mother, who was just standing there smiling, is now on her hands and knees with a totally different expression on her face. Better yet, she is making different noises than she had been. With a simple twist of the wrist, a seven-month-old has lightened the load in his hand, changed the color of the floor, changed his mother's posture, her facial expression, and the sounds she makes. No wonder he's fascinated! He has learned that he can do things to his environment that make it change substantially. Imagine the sense of mastery! You, however, are not pleased; in fact, you're terribly annoyed. You have every right to be, and expressing your annoyance is the best way for you to communicate clearly to your child that his behavior is totally unacceptable. But remember, if you can keep yourself sufficiently calm to remember anything, that your annoyed response is indeed confusing to your child, who is still absolutely fascinated by what he has just done. After all, he did not know that what he did was going to be judged unacceptable. So give your child another cup of milk. You know by now that he will surely try to spill the milk again. And this time he will look you straight in the face as he does spill it. At this instant, you will probably feel that your child is out to do you in. You may even wonder if he is destined to be a juvenile delinquent. Your feelings are all too understandable, but your child is concentrating not on your feelings but on finding out if the same twist of the wrist will again change the color of the floor, the posture of his mother, her facial expression, and the noises she makes. He wants to validate his hypothesis that the twist of his wrist caused the changes.

If you can understand how this common situation looks through your child's eyes, you can certainly understand his great urge to satisfy his curiosity. You have to realize that if you block his exploration completely, he may become even more fascinated and feel compelled to continue spilling things more often as a way to check his impact on his environment. If, on the other hand, you recognize his curiosity and understand his motivation, you can help channel his curiosity into a socially acceptable pattern. Try it this way.

By this time, your child has probably become fascinated with the fact that each time he twists his wrist what he releases from his cup always goes down and never up. He may have become interested in exploring the effects of gravity on released objects. So after making it clear that you will not tolerate his spilling milk, you can replace the cup with an object such as a rubber toy or wooden block, or, even better, a piece of crumpled newspaper. Show him that opening his hand and letting something like that drop makes you smile. Your smile indicates that he may drop those objects, but not his milk. In all likelihood, your child will continue to drop the newspaper until he is convinced that dropping it leads to a predictable set of events, specifically that it goes down and that making it go down is permissible in your eyes. After he's fully explored the matter of gravity and knows that objects of all sorts go down and not up, his curiosity will be satisfied. Now, since you have gotten across the idea that he cannot spill milk at the table, you can go on to teach him that there are times and places when it is permissible to spill a liquid. Let him play with water in his bath and spill it as much as he wants. Since he will quickly see that spilling water in the bath does not make you angry, he will play with it there until his curiosity about the mechanics of liquids is satisfied. The point of this whole example is that your child has a normal and natural curiosity which must be expressed. He requires your help and patience to satisfy it in a manner that it is neither dangerous nor destructive but is acceptable according to the rules and regulations you have set up. If you use discipline in this way, your child will learn what makes things happen, and he will also learn that what he does can elicit positive as well as negative responses in others. This is indeed a very useful lesson.

Some parents who find discipline difficult attempt to alter a child's environment to avoid having to say no, or otherwise restrict their child's behavior. They remove every object that might cause trouble and do all they can to outthink their child so that she never gets into a situation where she cannot behave just as she pleases. The child never gets taught to control herself because situations requiring that control never seem to arise. For example, it is crucially important that you prevent your child from shocking herself by putting her fingers or other objects into electrical outlets. One way to accomplish this is to cover up all the electric light outlets in your home. But it is far better to teach your child about electric outlets. You can do this the same way you teach a child not to tear magazines, that is, by reacting to her actions until she learns what is acceptable behavior. If you simply plug up the electrical outlets and avoid the problem, your child will never learn not to put her fingers in them. Ignorance like this can be harmful. Eventually your child will be in someone else's home where the electric outlets are not plugged up, and your child, not having learned not to put objects into outlets, may very well have an accident. What I am getting at is that you have to help your children learn what restrictions are and how to cope with them by themselves. If they do not experiment, they cannot learn. You do have to protect them from danger, but you must not protect them from learning.

When you discipline, be sure not to set limits that are too strict. Your child needs to explore the environment and satisfy his inquisitiveness. If your limits are overly constricting, you will stifle his curiosity. He may even grow to find learning an unpleasant process. Moreover, he may get so that he complies with any restriction, however absurd. He acts more like a polite robot than a happy child. Also when you discipline, remember to react positively to behavior you approve of as well as negatively to what you don't allow. Discipline is ineffective if your child feels you always say no. As your child accepts your discipline and learns to behave in a way that brings him approval, he will increase his sense of self-esteem from your favorable reactions and the reactions of others. He will be given the freedom to explore the world and at the same time feel protected. He will develop his own resources. Your child will not grasp discipline if you do not allow him to use his own resources in his efforts to cope with life's problems. Do not make the mistake of constantly doing things for your child. At the same time, help your child avoid the kind of overwhelming frustration that prevents him from having success in the first place.

I have often noticed the way parents deal with a child's homework, and it is a pretty good indication of the kind of parents they are. Basically, there are three types of parents when it comes to dealing with problems children face. One kind of parent is so geared to protecting his child from frustration that he sits down with his child each evening after dinner and essentially does his child's homework. Above all, he wants his child to get good grades and not be frustrated in the process. Then, there is the mother who not only insists that her child do his own homework immediately after school, but believes that stress is good for strengthening character. She adds lesson upon lesson to his homework load, thereby deliberately increasing his frustration and making it impossible for the child to feel that he has actually accomplished anything. This child often feels emotionally exhausted and overwhelmed. He is apt to be the kind of child who gives up, saying, "What's the use? Nothing I do satisfies her." Lastly, there is the parent who shows concern about her child's responsibility for doing his homework. She makes every effort to provide the most comfortable environment for doing homework, and she offers assistance in solving whatever problems arise. But under no circumstances does she actually do the homework for her child.

The effectiveness of the third kind of parent lies in her ability to help her son use his own resources for solving life's problems. This approach enriches a child's self-esteem, his feelings of responsibility, and his sense of individuality. Whether the problem is your ten-year-old's homework or your five-month-old reaching for a block, remember, don't take away your child's feeling of mastery by doing the job for him. Don't cause such stress and frustration that the pleasure is drained. Your child will only give up and never try again. Do help your child use his or her own resources to gain a sense of independence and individuality so that he can experience the great pleasure he will take in your pride in and your recognition of what he accomplished by himself—with your concerned assistance.

-XIII-

Changing Trends in Family Life

In recent years, substantial changes have taken place in family life. Needless to say, these changes have challenged the structure and even the existence of the traditional family, to say nothing of the traditional roles that various family members undertake. I believe that the nuclear family will survive, but an individual's motives for getting married and having a family will be quite different.

People are accepting the changing attitudes brought about by a lower birth rate, a growing divorce rate, and the increasing number of women who are moving away from household work and child rearing into the business or professional world. More young people decide not to marry at all, and many choose to structure family life so that it is based upon personal trust rather than legal or religious commitment. Since being divorced no longer carries the stigma of social failure, maintaining a bad marriage that has eroded over the years is no longer held in high esteem. More and more single people are attempting to raise children. Both men and women are moving into child rearing without a spouse. A few are successful; a lot are not. A number of single men are adopting children without taking on the responsibility of marriage, and some women who do not want to adopt a child are becoming pregnant by a man of their choice. They ask him simply to father their child and want no further commitment from him.

Society has begun to view sexual matters differently than in the past. There is increasing open-mindedness about sexual relations and technique, birth control, and abortion. More young people accept sexual encounters without the degree of emotional involvement that causes people to over-evaluate the importance of sex. In the past, forbidding sex and enforcing strict taboos made it more important than regarding it as a normal human need that requires expression for emotional and physical well-being. Sex is no longer available only in marriage; furthermore, the purpose for sexual activity is no longer primarily the production of children. Obviously this change is good for the children who are not born unwanted, since it increases the connection between marriage and children and diminishes the tie between marriage and sex. In short, sexual freedom has made sexual needs a bad reason for marriage and a worse reason for becoming pregnant.

Any challenge to the structure of the traditional family is bound to cause it to disintegrate where the structure was not very strong to begin with or where greater personal fulfillment for one of the individuals involved could only be obtained in other ways. The structure of the traditional family regarded the female as the caretaker of children and the home. For some women this was neither challenging nor sufficiently interesting to provide satisfaction. They began seeking their satisfactions outside the home. In years past, a woman's traditional role involved a large amount of work, some of it physical labor, and little time for boredom. Because their family duties could not be cared for by anyone else, they knew and felt they were essential. They actually did have responsibility for the survival of the family. In recent times this sense of purpose has disintegrated because mass production of household items has obsoleted the rewards of individual effort. The women's movement has successfully challenged the traditional family style that had come to offer little gratification to women. It forced both men and women to re-evaluate their roles to make them more meaningful to their ultimate purpose—gaining a feeling of importance for what they do. This challenge has led to much progress, for when institutions are challenged they either disintegrate because they are obsolete or become stronger by virtue of the challenge itself. Actually, it is my feeling that all the challenges to the traditional family, particularly those of the women's movement, will lead more people to greater fulfillment and therefore to an improvement in the quality of family life.

Another reason the traditional family began to disintegrate was that industry and government paid only lip service to the importance of family life. Taking on family responsibilities was exalted among the highest virtues and yet family responsibilities were, for the most part, ignored by the institutions of our society. Strange as it may sound, it was not the women's movement that most weakened the family and in the process taught women to seek satisfaction away from their homes, it was industry and government. I cannot tell you how many cases involving children with emotional problems include mothers who were overwhelmed by having to rear their children alone because the fathers were forced to be away. These fathers usually left their families not by choice but because they were sent off on long business trips by employers who disregarded the needs of that man's family. No effort was made to provide any opportunity for the family to travel together while the father was absent from home on business. Families, not just fathers, are uprooted periodically by job reassignments which convenience the employer—and in the process tear people away from relatives and friends, keep children from forming long-lasting relationships with other youngsters, cause difficulties in academic adjustment, and make wives feel less and less significant since they can do nothing but move along with their husbands when these job demands are made. Men who refused to accept these transfers lost their jobs or were not advanced in their companies. Wives could not effectively protest this since the livelihood of the family was at stake. Actually, it was not just the stress of the actual uprooting or the periodic estrangement of the father from his wife and children that eroded the family. Rather it was the overall attitude that everything else was more important than the family. Never did the employer concede that the needs of the family might come first. How ironic that the establishment has generally blamed our rebellious youth or the women's movement for the dissolution of the family. In fact, the neglect of the family by our institutions forced our young people to reevaluate their own goals in order to avoid the pitfalls they observed in their own families. When family needs were totally disregarded as fathers moved from place to place, the children took notice. They also noticed when fathers dedicated themselves for twenty or more years only to be let go as a result of two companies merging. The children, like the dedicated employee, became bitter. It was hard for them to see a man forty to forty-five years of age having so dedicated himself now unable to find another job because "who wants to hire a man at that stage in life?" It was precisely this kind of treatment that turned off many of our young people and led them to jobs and occupations that they thought would give them a chance to express their individuality away from an establishment that would certainly disregard their family needs and probably their own personal needs as well.

If we as a society are to strengthen the existence of the family, we as individuals must recognize the needs of each and every family member and expect society at large to recognize them too. Parenthood, in particular, must be given the prominence it deserves. People who take on that responsibility should be given the assistance they need to handle their family duties. If today's children are to grow into the responsible adults we hope they will be, it will be necessary to create the optimal conditions for their healthy emotional growth and development. To date, little has been done to provide flexible working hours for parents of children under the age of three; little effort has been made to accept family needs as being at least as important as the needs of industry or government; and little effort has been made to provide the kind of parent education that is necessary to prepare people for the enormous responsibility of bringing another human being into this world. Although we all know how important early influences are on later behavior, little has been done to prevent the development of emotional disorders and the criminal behavior, drug abuse, and child abuse that results. We simply do not offer the kind of environmental support required to counteract the development of emotional disturbances. Our society's disregard of the family has permeated all aspects of modern life, not because anyone fought to weaken the family but as a result of a blatant neglect of family needs, coupled with an overemphasis on the top priority of our respective vocations.

Changes in the structure of the traditional family have—not surprisingly—created new types of problems that require some consideration. For example, the single-parent experience. If it is indeed difficult and time consuming for two people to raise children successfully, it is obviously difficult for a single person. Any single person who plans to adopt a child or considers having one outside a total family experience should be fully aware of the tremendous commitment that this involves. Some people feel that simply having a child will make them, without further effort, at ease in parenthood. They're not always right. It is very easy to have a child, but it is extremely difficult to be a parent.

I am willing to grant that it may be better for a child to be cared for in the home of a single parent than to be raised in an institution that does not provide adequate time and attention. Nevertheless, I am inclined to discourage single parenthood. It always raises a question in my mind whether those people who deliberately decide to be single parents are doing so in the best interests of the child or for the satisfaction of some unknown or hidden self-interest. Not long ago I met a single man who was among the first legally to adopt a child. He obviously glorified parenthood and was convinced he could adequately cope with all its demands as he continued living the way he always had. As it turned out, the child he adopted was hyperactive. His son got into all kinds of trouble and required special care and education. As his problems mounted, this man began to become overwhelmed. In the beginning he unconsciously rejected his son and later on actively rejected him. Clearly, the child needed help. Although his adoptive father had had all the best intentions, he hadn't foreseen anything but his own desire to be a single parent. He related to that and not the realities of having responsibility for a child. He saw the pleasures but not the problems. Eventually, he had to seek professional help to cope with his feelings of rejecting the child he initially desired.

With less stigma attached to divorces, the divorced-parent experience has become very common. In fact, I myself have come to recognize that many divorces are not a sign of failure, but of success. In the past, many very poor marriages which caused tension and pressure for all members of the family tended to persist, either because divorce was regarded as a disgrace or because a divorce was impossible to obtain. Often when an unsuccessful marriage drags on, everyone involved suffers. Divorce as an end to such a destructive situation can be a positive experience for everyone, even though the transition will cause tremendous stresses. As we all know, divorces are particularly stressful on children but not, in my opinion, always so stressful as to warrant, for that reason alone, the continuation of a worthless marriage. With proper parental support, a child can be helped through the experience and often ends up happier than if the marriage continued. If society really meant what it says about making divorces easier on children, a great deal of revamping should take place in the existing marital law. Antiquated legal notions of what is best for children must be reexamined, and family law should be substantially modified to prevent children from being used as hostages by either parent when a marriage breaks up. The legal procedures should be modified so that men are given equal consideration. To date, the courts generally regard women as more able to care for children than men. This is by no means always the case. In fact, there are tremendous numbers of men who make more effective parents than women. If the best interests of children were really of concern, it would seem only fair to base arrangements for the care of the children of divorced parents on the relative abilities of the parents to meet the needs of the child. It cannot possibly help any child to make this decision solely on the basis of the parent's gender. Personally, I believe that until laws are changed to acknowledge the rights of children in the matter of their parents' divorces, children will be exploited and suffer unnecessarily when marriages break up. Society ought also to know that to get fathers more involved in the responsibilities of child rearing, it will have to give them equal rights with mothers in the event of divorce.

With the changing trends in family life, I believe strongly in encouraging more and more people to consider seriously having no children at all. Generally speaking, many people who do not have children are bombarded by family and friends who react as if there were something inherently wrong in being married and not having children. I admire people who give very careful thought to the responsibilities of parenthood, the demands of their work, and their responsibilities to each other, and then decide not to have children. They are certainly more thoughtful, less selfish, and more responsible than the person who blindly conceives a child without knowing what is in store. Too often this type of parent finds out that "this is not what I had in mind." Far too many people have thoughtlessly allowed themselves to get involved in parenthood, only to find that they lack the temperament and motivation to devote themselves sufficiently to their children. I have often heard couples who remained childless called "selfish." To me it is far more selfish to bring children into this world and then have someone else rear them. Happily, many people absolutely flourish in the role of parent, at the same time providing their children with an ideal environment for emotional health. If we can only liberate people from the idea that they must grow up, get married, and have children, we would be free to make our choices based upon our capabilities. We must encourage our young people to consider alternatives to parenthood early enough so that they can plan for them. If, having planned for these alternatives, they still choose to be parents, they will have chosen positively, not passively. If more people are encouraged to consider the alternative of not having any children at all, then other people can be free to have as many children as they desire and are capable of rearing effectively, without worrying about the consequences of population growth.

Many couples who choose to have a child are immediately encouraged to have a second child. The pressure, often great pressure, usually comes in the form of implications that an only child will be a spoiled child or that an only child will grow up to be lonely. Beware of this pressure! The number of children you have is a personal decision, yours and yours alone. Being an only child does not cause hardship. If all you care to have is one child, then have one, and do not have any more. If you convince yourself that you are having a second child simply to provide companionship for your first, you might end up disliking parenthood, yourself, and both children as well. I can assure you that for each only child I have ever met who wished he had a brother or sister, I know of one who was delighted to be alone.

In preparing for parenthood, I think it is important to consider where parenthood will fit in the total structure of your life. What are you going to do after your child-rearing years are over? Many people obtain, and quite properly so, a great deal of self-esteem in their parenthood. Some have few alternatives for gaining the same kind of satisfaction. Many of these parents cling to their children after their children are grown up. It is as if the parents are afraid of having their children leave home. They tend to infantalize their children, over-protect them, and keep them dependent for as long as possible. For example, as the distraught mother of a teen-ager complained that her daughter was keeping bad company and was in danger of getting into trouble, I sensed the mother's dependence on her daughter. Whenever I tried to get her to describe her daughter's problems or the specific things she feared, this mother became defensive, vague, and evasive. She really related only to her fears of her daughter's possible problems and not to her daughter. It was as if she needed to construct problems in her own mind to justify her insistence that her daughter stay close to her and continue to live at home.

Needless to say, when your children are grown and living away from home, you may find yourself under stress. You may notice depression and a feeling of worthlessness which may lead you to impose yourself on your children in a way that makes you a burden to them and intensifies their wish to get away from you and be on their own. When examining these situations, I often find parents who have had unsuccessful marriages or marital problems they have never had to face because they have immersed themselves in the role of mother or father to de-emphasize their role as husband or wife. Needless to say, when being a mother or father becomes less significant in that person's life, he or she begins to have to face the problems of the marriage. There are also parents aware of their marital problems who have elected to stay together because of their children. For them, the end of the child-rearing years is also the end of the marriage. I sincerely feel that the changing trends in family life will make it possible for more people to prepare themselves more effectively for the end of parenthood. I feel that this will come about partly by encouraging young people to prepare themselves for active business and professional lives so that they need not feel a loss of self-esteem when the tasks of child rearing are over. In this way, the end of parenthood will involve a quantitative shift in the distribution of one's time rather than a qualitative shift in one's life which in some cases has been extremely difficult to make and in other cases impossible.

In the future, more people will be entering marital relationships with greater understanding of themselves and the responsibilities of family life. Fewer people will be forced into taking on the role of parenthood. Clearly this will contribute toward making marriages of higher quality. Likewise, children can only benefit from the new realignment of the relationship between sex and marriage and parenthood. Sex and marriage and children are no longer synonymous. We are slowly, and I think wisely, beginning to grasp the idea that marriage is primarily for children. As we increasingly accept this concept, we will evaluate possible spouses in terms of their parenthood potential. I think this is all to the good since I am convinced that the nuclear family is still the best way to raise children, particularly from the child's point of view. The nuclear family provides a structure where a child of either gender can experience close relationships with adults of each gender who share responsibilities and who also provide a child with an opportunity to relate to these same individuals. Children can see a mother and father expressing love and affection, and also anger and annoyance. A child can learn to come to terms with his various emotional reactions from the model set in the nuclear family. In this way he can learn to express his feelings and also to respect the feelings of others.

Children are the future of humankind. Our hopes for peace, for scientific advance, and for responsible leadership are in their hands. This is why I consider parenthood one of the most important tasks a person can undertake, not only for himself and his children but for society in general. If our civilization is to survive, we must offer our offspring the opportunity to develop a sense of individuality, achieve a sense of self-esteem, be capable of making decisions rationally, and above all to establish the kind of trusting and close relationships with other human beings which enables them to express a sense of love.

Index